BECOMING WHOLE

How to Prevent Stockholm Syndrome and Transcend Darkness in Your Life and Relationships

MEREDITH MILLER

Post Hill Press

A POST HILL PRESS BOOK
ISBN: 979-8-89565-098-1
ISBN (eBook): 979-8-89565-099-8

Becoming Whole:
How to Prevent Stockholm Syndrome and Transcend Darkness in Your Life and Relationships

Cover design by Cody Corcoran

Meredith Miller is not a medical doctor or therapist. She does not diagnose or treat disease. She does not give medical advice nor make claims or promises of curing any illness or disease. Your reliance upon information and content obtained by you at or through this publication is solely at your own risk. This holistic work is about expanding self-awareness, empowerment and liberation in order to thrive in your life and relationships. Thank you for taking responsibility for yourself.

Post Hill Press
New York • Nashville
posthillpress.com

Published in the United States of America
1 2 3 4 5 6 7 8 9 10

To proclaim liberty to the captives, and the opening of the prison to those who are bound.

Isaiah 61:1

TABLE OF CONTENTS

PART TWO: THE LIBERATION OF SOULS

INTRODUCTION

Many people wonder why they stayed so long in an abusive relationship or situation, or why one of their loved ones did.

Likewise, in the early 2020s, people have been wondering why so many others complied with tyranny and abuse on a global scale, and why they couldn't see what was happening.

It's much easier to ask these questions from the outside or in retrospect. When you're in it, it's difficult to fully understand what's happening and how you're participating. You feel like you can't do anything to change your life circumstances, so you adapt to survive them.

The reason why people stay and cooperate in horrible situations and relationships has nothing to do with intelligence or education level. In other words, it's not that they're stupid.

After delivering more than 5,000 hours of one-on-one private and group coaching, I've met very smart people who fell into psychologically abusive relationships. I've also met highly educated people who had abusive partners. I've even worked with therapists, psychologists (some with PhDs!), and psychiatrists who ended up in abusive marriages and didn't recognize the abuse, or get out for years or decades, despite their professional education and intelligence.

Likewise, most of the world's doctors, psychologists, therapists, psychiatrists, religious leaders, and spiritual teachers have passively or actively enabled the tyranny, isolation, coercion, abuse, and segregation of individuals in society since 2020.

The majority of leaders and practitioners in those industries—the very people who have been trained to understand the nature of the body, mind, spirit, and health of human beings—didn't see what was happening through the lens of their craft.

Here we are, several years later, with so much evidence coming out, yet some people are still justifying why tyranny was a *necessary evil*, while minimizing or erasing the harm, as if the crimes against humanity didn't happen. Many people are pretending like nothing happened.

It's shocking but not surprising. This is how abusive social systems work, from families to workplaces, communities, and society. The collective fantasy is contagious. The primary contagion is a mind virus.

I have compassion for those going through abuse because I know what it's like to fall into victimhood, to cooperate and comply with abusers, becoming an enabler of my own captivity. I was in that state of consciousness for decades, not knowing there was a way out. It was just life. It didn't look like war or a hostage situation on the outside, which is why it was so confusing that my inner experience was as if it were.

A few years ago, a Hinge date led me to a conversation with a man around my age from Iran. He told me, "This, what you call *trauma*, this is just life." He grew up during the Iran–Iraq war in the 1980s when bombs were hitting just blocks away. Most of us in the West are fortunate not to know what it's like to live like that. Yet in some way, we've all had experiences in which we sensed imminent death, though not necessarily literally.

At a neurological level, the physiological and psychological sense of danger and life threat are the same. The *perception* of the experience becomes the reality.

Humans have innate survival mechanisms built into the nervous system that help us to adapt in order to get through whatever life brings to our personal experience. We cohabit in partnerships, friendships, families, and communities where our nervous systems communicate based on our programming. Our adaptations to life seem to biologically, psychologically, and spiritually dance with each other's to the tune of our unresolved trauma. This happens automatically, without our awareness.

The conscious mind, what we are aware of, is only about 10 percent of our consciousness. That's where education, information, knowledge and training are stored.

The other 90 percent is the subconscious—what we aren't aware of. Most of what we do is driven by the subconscious, including our reaction to other people and life in general. This can include repressed feelings, emotions, and implicit memories as well as our programming.

The subconscious gets programmed from conception throughout our lifetime, most especially during childhood. We also inherit subconscious programs from our ancestors and the collective consciousness.

The subconscious mind can appear to be elusive and hidden, though it can be accessed through the body, which is visible and tangible. The body *is* the subconscious, as neuroscientist Candace Pert discovered.

The body and behavior always tell the story. The issues we have with our bodies, and the behaviors that are sabotaging our lives, are connected to the repressed and reactive themes of emotion and energy in the subconscious. Unaware of this connection, we can feel like victims of happenstance instead of owning the power of being co-creators of our reality.

The mechanisms built into the human brain and nervous system for survival can end up working against us. On the one hand, these help us to survive intensely stressful experiences when there's no escape. On the other hand, these are the core underlying factors that set people up to fall into abusive relationships and tyranny, then continue cooperating and complying because it feels like there's no way out.

This is what happened in 2020 when all things COVID began to flip our world upside down.

The very mechanisms that are intended to keep us alive through self-preservation can also cause dysfunction, disconnection and *dis-ease* in life. These survival mechanisms have always been part of our human condition. Yet, in recent years, these mechanisms have become terribly amplified and distorted by global crises.

This book is about the state of captivity and the liberation of souls. It will help you to understand how Stockholm syndrome happens in real life, how you can prevent it, and how you can transcend the darkness in your life and relationships in order to restore wholeness and freedom. Stockholm syndrome is far more common than you might think. It's less about falling in love with your captors, and more about the state of consciousness that is captivity, and what people do to adapt and survive it.

Why am I writing and speaking about these topics? I know this state of consciousness well. I lived most of my life in it without realizing I was captive to my programming.

For several years before 2020, I thought I was finally free and living my best life. In a way I was, certainly much more than I had been during the first three-plus decades of my life. But also, not really. Deep down, I still had these programs of captivity. I wasn't really free within the constraints of the life I had designed for myself, which, ironically, was intended to give me a sense of freedom. I was still avoiding and escaping the unresolved past.

I discovered that after the plandemic began and the world locked down into a state of captivity. The collective trauma brought to the surface the places in me that weren't liberated or empowered. So, I went back in the trenches. It wasn't planned, but it was a calling. I had to re-live it, at another level, so I could guide people to another level.

In recent years, through observing myself and how people were responding around the world, I was able to understand that state of consciousness more deeply and gained valuable new insights. We'll explore the holistic micro-to-macro patterns of captivity and liberation in this book.

We've all had certain pain points touched and triggered by the events of recent years. For each of us, it's relative to our personal and ancestral patterns as well as how we are dealing with our own trauma in general. Most people don't recognize the gravity of what happened since 2020 because they're also in denial about their own unresolved past. It's very common to suppress, avoid, and numb our pain in order to escape it.

I will give you an incisive look at the patterns beneath the surface in abusive relationships and social systems, such as families or workplaces, and especially what happened in society in the early 2020s that led most of the world into a state of captivity and compliance. By the end of this book, you'll gain new perspectives of how these themes are all connected and why they are coming to a head now. We are living in a pivotal moment in human history. Where we go from here depends on what we do.

Part One of this book is an exploration of why people comply and cooperate with abuse. It explains how we can end up (unknowingly) enabling the abusers and get trapped in a state of captivity, which can last long after leaving the abusive relationship or situation.

A state of captivity is induced through four specific parameters, which have always been used for the control of domestic violence victims as well as in abusive families, workplaces, cults, and society at large:

1. Isolation (physical, psychological, or both),
2. Acts of perceived kindness,
3. Perceived threat to one's life, and
4. Perceived inability to escape.

These are the same four parameters that induce Stockholm syndrome, otherwise known as trauma bonding, traumatic entrapment, or appeasement. These terms all describe the same phenomenon, whether it happens between strangers, with loved ones in intimate partnerships and family, in workplaces, religious and spiritual communities, or even in society. The behavioral result is compliance, and the state of consciousness is captivity.

Each parameter will be explored in its own chapter, including specific examples that you'll be able to relate to experiences that you may have had in your personal life, or through observing what has happened in the world.

You'll see exactly why each (and all) of these parameters must happen in order to induce such a state of captivity in the target. You'll gain an understanding of how the same patterns are present from the interpersonal to the societal level due to our human survival adaptations.

By dissecting these parameters and looking at the big picture, you can strengthen your awareness in order to identify any areas of vulnerability to emotional manipulation. The more able you are to recognize these patterns in real life, from the micro level to the macro level, the more likely you'll be able to prevent it in the future.

Unfortunately, the concept of Stockholm syndrome and trauma bonding is greatly misunderstood by the institutions of psychology and psychiatry, two industries that function much like cults. Each has its governing board, which controls the licensing—the ability to practice and earn a livelihood—of all those who invested years of study and work, and often a small fortune, to hold such a license. One must subscribe to the ideology of Big Pharma (in psychiatry) and the dominant political bias (in psychology) in order to not be ostracized, smeared, threatened, and penalized.

Over the years, I've heard some psychiatrists and psychologists say that Stockholm syndrome can't apply to psychological abuse in relationships because it must occur between strangers in a situation of physical confinement.

They're looking at it entirely too literally.

After decades of observing these patterns in myself and others—and seeing the striking similarities from one relationship or social system to the next—I have come to understand that this is part of the human condition. Stockholm syndrome can happen whether there's physical confinement or not. That's why I've renamed this state of consciousness *state of captivity*.

My perspective of this topic comes from a holistic lens because body–mind–spirit is the paradigm in which I work as holistic coach. I am not a psychologist, therapist, psychiatrist, or doctor. I do not diagnose diseases or provide medical advice. I do not subscribe to any particular dogma or school of thought. My vision encompasses an expanded perspective of what it means to be human, rather than being influenced by a top-down protocol of industry consensus and ideology, or the pixelated and fragmented model of the human being that we find in modern medicine.

This book does not make scientific claims, though I cite some scientific studies that support my perspectives. What I am offering is a holistic view of what happened during the early 2020s, where we are now, and where we can go from here.

Healing and evolution are an art, not a science. You could study these processes through a lens of science, and you might discover some interesting and fascinating things, but you'll miss the essence. My aim with this work is to touch the human essence.

I am not trying to improve the old model, which clearly isn't working. My work on this topic aims to inspire a new perspective of the human condition, from the micro level to the macro level, and the power that we have to participate in our own captivity or liberate our souls in order to co-create the life we want to live.

The state of captivity is an *inner* state. It is psychological, neurological, and spiritual. Therefore, it's a *psycho-neuro-spiritual* state of captivity. It's a state of consciousness that becomes reality.

The subconscious mind cannot differentiate between what's vividly imagined and what's actually happening. Physical confinement isn't required because there's a *perception* of no escape, and that's what matters to the subconscious, which drives our behavior. While the prison bars may be imaginary, they are very real to those who are experiencing them.

For example, victims of domestic violence (including psychological abuse) will often leave the house multiple times a day. They keep going back to the abusive environment of the home because they *believe* they can't leave that relationship or situation.

What's keeping them there is not usually physical force or constraint. It's something else.

For most of my life, I was free to move around, yet my soul wasn't free. I was trapped in the state of captivity, which would get transferred from one relationship or situation to the next. It was even happening when I was alone.

All abusers and tyrants want others to comply with their every whim. They aim to exert dominance and control over their targets. This is most effective when the target has the illusion of freedom.

What we are witnessing on the macro level in society are the same patterns of narcissistic abuse that happen in family systems and interpersonal relationships. This form of abuse is predominantly psychological (mental and emotional) and spiritual, though it can involve elements of other forms of abuse as well (financial, sexual, technological, and physical).

It's important to know that it doesn't just go away with time. Once a person escapes an abusive situation or relationship, the state of captivity is still active in the mind, body, and soul. People can spend a whole lifetime locked in that state of consciousness, unable to break free and heal, while not understanding what's happening or how they're participating in their own captivity.

That's also why it's possible to be aware of the abuse and tyranny that's taking place in our world, while not being liberated, empowered, or healed from it.

One might wonder how tyrants could get so many individuals—even billions of people in a global society—to comply. It's actually quite simple.

Eventually, due to the ongoing intensity of the psychological and spiritual warfare over time, the target ends up in a state of learned helplessness and spiritual bankruptcy. When all hope is lost, the only thing left is emptiness. That's where a person becomes powerless, helpless, and hopeless, retreating into debility, dependence, dread, and apathy.

This is the state of consciousness that leads to escapism and compliance as survival mechanisms. And that's exactly where perpetrators aim to keep their targets, whether individuals or entire societies.

The same tactics are being copied and pasted from one social crisis to the next, whether for war or genocide; the economy; the poisoning of the air, water, and food; public health and individual healthcare; the climate change narrative; digital control systems; or more "pandemics." They are all used to drive people toward a desired outcome of learned helplessness and compliance.

We are already being ushered into the next frontier of captivity through technological and artificial intelligence (AI) developments and their integration into nearly every aspect of human life. COVID-19 was merely a stepping stone on the way to this technocratic digital slavery system that we are speeding toward at warp speed.

First, we need to understand the problem—how we got here—in order to see new solutions, opportunities, and possibilities of where we can go now as individuals and humanity. Like Dante Alighieri, we are being called to take a journey through the darkness of *Inferno,* in order to climb back up through *Purgatorio*, so we can rise into *Paradiso*.

Part Two of this book is about the liberation of souls. Many of us have been through existentially shattering experiences in recent years at the personal level—and much of society has been shattered at the collective level. The impact of these events has affected every aspect of human life. *Our relationship with existence has been shattered since 2020.*

We'll explore how we can use these unsettling times for post-traumatic growth. The disruptive crises are offering us an opportunity to make new choices with renewed perspective so we can create the life we want to live instead of drifting on automaton mode deeper into captivity. We are in a precarious position. It's also an incredible invitation to evolve. What matters is what we do with the invitation.

According to the National Domestic Violence Hotline, domestic violence victims return to their abusers an average of seven times.[1]

From my observations, it's not always the same abuser. What usually happens is people fall into additional abusive relationships and situations, each time thinking this is *finally* the answer to their problems.

The same trend occurs on the macro level in society. When we learn to recognize what's happening and do the inner work so we can make new choices, then we can create another way of living and being. Otherwise, history will continue repeating itself and this will become the burden that we pass on to the next generations, like those who came before us.

Yet this time the stakes are much higher. We are currently at the precipice of the amplification of our unresolved past, mirrored back to us through AI because humans are creating technology in their image.

I will provide some holistic perspectives as well as tactical practices for becoming whole by liberating your soul from the state of captivity, integrating the trauma, restoring your light, and building resilience in the 2020s. I will also encourage you to see that it's possible to thrive after these experiences, using the adversity as an opportunity for personal evolution, which will have a positive effect on yourself, the world around you, and future generations.

Trauma fragments us. Not just psychologically, but energetically—disrupting our connection to self, to others, to God, to life itself. We begin to live from protective and defensive adaptations instead of presence and wholeness.

That's why my work is called *Inner Integration.*

I use the word *integration* throughout this book to describe the process of reclaiming what trauma once severed: our connection, coherence and truth.

In mainstream psychology, the word "integration" often refers to the process of incorporating fragmented parts of the psyche into a more cohesive whole. This is a helpful foundation—but in the context of trauma healing and deep soul work, I'm speaking in a broader, multi-dimensional sense.

Integration isn't simply about putting pieces back together. It's about metabolizing what once overwhelmed and collapsed us. It's about transforming what was once held in separation—memories, emotions, beliefs, thoughtforms, identities—into coherence, presence, and deeper wholeness.

Integration isn't about erasing what happened. It's about changing our relationship with what happened, so it no longer defines us, distorts us, or disrupts our capacity to live from essence.

To integrate doesn't mean to "fix" or forget what happened. It's also not about going back to who we were before. It means to allow what was once exiled—emotionally, mentally, energetically, and spiritually—to return in a new form.

Integration is the alchemy of turning fragmentation into embodiment. It's not theoretical. It's visceral.

To integrate the past is to reclaim the parts of ourselves that were frozen in pain, exiled by shame, or dissociated by fear. It's the sacred work of digesting what was too much to feel at the time, so that the body and soul no longer need to carry it in shadow or silence. This creates the space for something new.

To integrate after trauma is to break free from the repetitive loops, to stop living in reaction to what happened, and to begin living in alignment with what now wants to emerge.

Integration is how we transmute the residue of survival programs into the radiance of wholeness. This book is an invitation into that process of *becoming whole*. From this state, we are free to create, connect, and contribute from our deepest truth.

We are living in wild and pivotal years on planet Earth, a culmination of centuries or perhaps millennia of abuse, trauma, and crises. I believe that those of us who are alive now were born for these times.

Can we integrate the past so that we can create a new future?

This is the evolutionary calling of our lifetime. How we respond as individuals will determine our personal fate, and the sum of our individual choices will become the future of humanity—the legacy that we pass on.

PART ONE

THE STATE OF CAPTIVITY

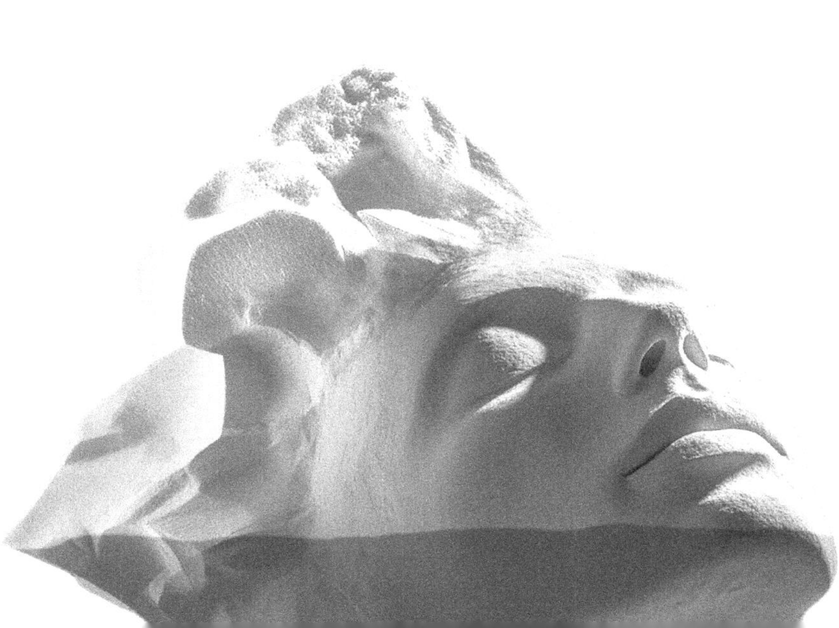

CHAPTER 1
PARAMETER ONE

Isolation

The first thing an abuser does is to start isolating the target from other people and outside perspectives in order to distort and control information and reality.

The goal of the isolation is for the target to become fully subscribed to the perpetrator's narrative. The key is that the target has no access to information that contradicts what the abuser wants the target to believe.

The abuser positions him or herself as the only trustworthy source of what's real, good, and true—devaluing, distorting, and discarding all information, perspectives, and people who contradict the abuser's narrative.

This is how the abuser becomes the center of information and communication in an abusive system like a family, workplace, or other social group. All members are trained to look to the abuser to define reality and the narrative of the group, as well as the role of each individual. Independent thinking is discouraged, shamed, and penalized.

The narrative of reality becomes like a hypnotic trance. This is highly contagious in a social system, creating a type of collective trance, which all members are tuned into through the group environment.

The abuser's enablers in the system will support and spread the acceptable narrative. Many will do this unintentionally without realizing how they're participating as "flying monkeys." Others willingly sacrifice their integrity and conscience because they depend on the abuser in some way—that could be for money, status, emotional support, physical security, living situation, or their very livelihood.

The enablers maintain the abusive system and the narrative. This is why everyone in the cult will turn against you if you challenge the abuser's narrative. It's also why you'll need to look for support outside the family or other abusive social system if you want to stay sane and leave the toxic environment.

Isolation can be physical or psychological

Physical isolation could involve situations of confinement where the target is forced to stay in a certain location, such as in a hostage situation.

In overt abusive relationships, targets may be threatened to stay in a particular place—including their own home—and not permitted to see other people by use of force, threat, or intimidation *for their own good.*

In covert abusive situations, the emotional manipulator will use more subtle ways of getting the target to voluntarily stay home or isolate from loved ones. Manipulators often use fear propaganda, such as saying that the target's family or friends are trying to destroy their relationship, or that they said things they didn't say, or that other people are somehow dangerous. This includes telling you that you can't trust your friends and family because they don't want the best for you. Meanwhile the covert abuser is positioned as the only one who cares about you.

The most sophisticated covert types usually get their targets to consent to the isolation by believing it's their own idea or truly for their own good. They'll tell you it's for your protection; it's because they care and want you to be safe.

With physical isolation, there is an element of social distancing. It's interesting that that was the exact phrase used in the 2020 government campaign to get people to stay home and keep six feet apart.

Isolation could be physical confinement, but most people in abusive relationships leave the house every day to go to work, take the kids to school and activities, go to the grocery store—and they continue to return home. This is why it's important to understand the impact of psychological isolation.

Psychological isolation is a way of separating people emotionally and mentally from their family and friends, even if they're in physical or virtual contact. When you're afraid to talk about controversial topics, or you don't perceive reality in the same way as those surrounding you, or you feel like no one else understands you, that causes feelings of psychological isolation. This is why you can be surrounded by people and still feel lonely or isolated.

The impact of prolonged isolation, whether physical or psychological, makes it difficult for the target to get help or even to ask for help.

The distortion of reality

The result of the isolation is the total domination of the target's reality. Gaslighting is the main tool used to isolate the target.

Gaslighting is the distortion of the perception of reality to the point where the target may even doubt his or her own sanity or memory. The abuser edits and erases history, even things you saw or heard with your own eyes and ears in order to make you doubt your perception of what's really happening.

It can be overt, for example when the abuser says, "That didn't happen" right after something clearly happened.

It can also be covert, through an insidious, meticulous, and subtle, ongoing campaign to get the target to doubt that what he or she sees and hears is real.

The distortion of reality is also accomplished through covert-aggressive tactics, such as smear campaigns, triangulation, and stonewalling. Outside perspectives are devalued and dismissed, often through *ad hominem* attacks on a person's character. A wedge is driven between the target and anyone with a divergent perspective. Serious conversations about accountability and resolution are avoided and thwarted.

It could appear to be easier for abusers to dominate and control the perception of reality in an interpersonal relationship, family system, workplace, or cult. You might wonder how, in 2020, it was possible to psychologically isolate the entire world and lock us into a particular narrative.

Small businesses were forced to close. Many of us found ourselves at corporate grocery stores, walking through the aisles as messages were being played on the loudspeakers, bombarding our subconscious while we were shopping. Government, corporations, and the complicit media reminded us to stay six feet apart, to wear a mask, and to stay home and order delivery or contactless pick-up.

In 2021, the messages focused on getting vaccinated, a service that many of the corporate stores offered on site, for your convenience. Yet the term "vaccine" is another distortion of reality. The definition of "vaccination" was changed by the U.S. Centers for Disease Control and Prevention (CDC) in the post-COVID era—from the act of producing immunity, to producing *protection*, from a specific disease—and the mRNA genetic technology is completely different than what we've always known as vaccines. I will use the terms vax, vaxxed, and unvaxxed in this book purposefully in order not to legitimize or normalize this distortion.

We have seen extensive control of public information, especially online. *Information control is reality control.*

In this case, there was a technological delivery of the perpetrator's messaging. While everyone was forced to stay home, people turned to social media to feel a sense of connection. Propaganda was pushed on those sites, relentlessly bombarding us with repetitive language and imagery. Extensive censorship took place to control information.

Much of the internet has been erased since 2020. You might have noticed that it became difficult to use search engines and get relevant information instead of highly curated search results that end after a page or two. If you didn't save the URL of news articles or other sites where you found information contradicting the Official Narrative, it became almost impossible to find those pages again. Viral videos with alternative information were often taken down in a matter of days or hours.

People were used as pawns to spread the narrative through their online social networks, much like how people in any abusive family or social system are used as enablers to promote the abuser's narrative. The deployment of social media was essential for narrative control.

In any abusive relationship, the perpetrator will repeat key phrases, often inventing new definitions of words. Most of the mainstream media around the world were pushing the narrative in lockstep, translating the key lingo into the world's languages. I speak five languages and verified this with my own eyes and ears.

Each of those key terms—quarantine, social distancing, stay six feet (two meters) apart, asymptomatic transmission, stay home and save lives, safe and effective—were repeated incessantly and used in combination with emotionally provoking images and videos to brainwash the public. Each word or phrase came with its own zip file–type of "download," which instantly evoked the corresponding imagery, emotions, and feelings from the subconscious, which then triggered the desired behavioral response.

Likewise, the symptoms of COVID-19 were described and repeated incessantly with strong imagery through hypnotic rhythms, creating suggestions for the subconscious mind.

"Watch out, you'll catch a terrible disease," Joseph Murphy wrote in his 1963 book *The Power of Your Subconscious Mind.* "Symptoms of almost any disease can be induced in hypnotic subjects by suggestion. For example, a subject in the hypnotic state can develop a high temperature, flushed face or chills according to the nature of the suggestion given."[2]

Social media platforms were complicit in promoting the Official Narrative by pushing government-sponsored campaigns, deleting and shadow-banning posts, or disqualifying posts with numerous "fact-checkers" sponsored by corporations doing the bidding of governments. One of the posts I made on Facebook in 2020 had *seven* different tags by the thought police, a.k.a. fact-checkers.

People who dared to have a different opinion or question the Official Narrative were shamed, mocked, attacked, and minimized through smear campaigns. We were told it's because we're not experts and we should only listen to "trusted sources." Newspaper headlines were frequently emphasized with the qualifier "experts say." Public officials told us they would determine who the trusted sources are, and we should outsource our thinking to them because *they know better than us*. Said every abuser, ever.

When brave doctors and scientists spoke up instead of parroting the Official Narrative like the rest of their colleagues, they were silenced and smeared. Many even had their medical licenses threatened or revoked. When doctors are being censored during a pandemic, *Houston we have a problem*.

Yet most people didn't notice or care because they had already outsourced their power and critical thinking to the authorities. We were told to obey the medical system that was long ago socially engineered to groom people into surrendering the responsibility for their health to medical authorities.

Information about early and alternative medical treatments and prevention was suppressed and discarded. People (including doctors) who dared to use alternative medicine that wasn't on the officially approved list or those who spoke up about the medical assault taking place in hospitals by way of the harmful top-down protocols that were implemented were smeared, threatened, and demonized. As interdisciplinary researcher Denis Rancourt has exposed, "Within the present state of knowledge, it is possible that the declared Covid pandemic (2020-2023) was entirely caused by the coordinated and largescale mandates, measures, so-called responses, and medical assaults including testing, diagnostic bias, isolation, denial of treatment (especially antibiotics for pneumonia), mechanical ventilation, sedation, experimental and improper treatments, and vaccination."[3]

According to doctors I've spoken with, there is a long tradition in medicine of physicians sharing information and questioning the use of treatments and medications. Doctors used to be able to discuss such issues together as professionals. They were allowed to explore treatment options rather than being forced to follow a protocol from above and prohibited from questioning or disobeying those top-down orders.

One doctor told me that in more than twenty-five years of working in medicine, she never saw such anger and hostility from her colleagues as she did when she or anyone else questioned the efficacy or safety of COVID "vaccines."

Even now, several years later, at gatherings of global organizations, we hear public figures openly calling for more censorship and information control. In early 2023, when most people assumed the pandemic was over, an entire segment of the elite gathering at Davos was dedicated to "the danger of misinformation," a group of powerful people that is still pushing the "safe and effective" lie.

The person (or people) controlling the information determines how others perceive reality. Most people are not psychologically strong enough to maintain their perception of reality when consistently contradicted by the group. We are biologically wired to seek safety in the herd. It's a miracle when a person is able to own his reality when everyone else turns against him or insists that he's wrong.

It's often only one or a few people in an extended abusive family system who wake up. As soon as they start speaking the truth about the abuse, everyone else turns on them in order to maintain the status quo.

People will usually protect the image of the family or abuser(s) because that's where they get their distorted sense of safety and reality. Most people identify so deeply with their family, political party, religion, ethnicity, or social group that any critical view of the whole is interpreted as a personal attack threatening their existence.

In 2020, people in many areas around the world were subjected to domestic confinement under threat of arrest and police brutality. These brutal acts took place across America and other countries, many of which were shown on the news and social media platforms. The traumatic imagery of those videos encouraged others to comply, reminding them what would happen if they didn't.

In some places with a recent history of tyranny and dictatorship, such as Spain—where *franquismo* ended in 1975—citizens took part in collective COVID rituals, such as standing on their balconies at 8 p.m. to clap for the health workers. Those who didn't show up on their balconies to join in were sometimes reported to hotlines by their neighbors. People were also not allowed to receive visits from friends or romantic partners. Many neighbors reported those who violated this mandate.

Yet even in America, *the land of the free*, some governors and mayors encouraged people to report businesses that were open so they could cut off their utilities. Others threatened to hunt down people for disobeying the domestic confinement orders.

New York City had hotlines for reporting people who violated the lockdown mandates. Thankfully there were some citizens who could see the insanity of these tyrannical measures. Prank phone calls were made to those numbers. Memes went around the internet nicknaming those the 1-800-IM-A-NAZI hotlines.

There were many spectacular divide-and-conquer tactics among We the People to make us see each other as the enemy instead of uniting together as the human race against tyranny. One way or another, most of us fell right into that trap.

The downstream effects of isolation

Social isolation creates a state of disconnection. The human (mammalian) autonomic nervous system (ANS) reads disconnection as dangerous or life threatening because we are social creatures and we rely on the herd for survival.

Connection is our biological imperative, as professor of psychiatry and creator of the Polyvagal Theory, Dr. Stephen Porges, emphasizes in his work.

Through *neuroception*, a term coined by Dr. Porges, the ANS is constantly scanning the environment for cues of safety and threat. When it perceives isolation, that is interpreted as unsafe, which then triggers the defense system. That's why the sense of danger or life threat evokes the survival mechanisms of fight, flight, freeze, and fawn.

Neuroscientist Dr. Andrew Huberman cites scientific literature in his podcast showing that prolonged isolation causes humans to become more irritable and aggressive toward others when given a chance to connect again.[4]

We have seen escalating domestic and public violence and aggression in recent years. Many people are noticing this while driving and at public gatherings, and, of course, online. Due to the uptick in these behaviors, some airports now have signs warning passengers that violence and aggression will not be tolerated.

In that same podcast episode, Dr. Huberman explains that prolonged isolation has devastating consequences on mammals, including humans, causing chronically elevated stress hormones. This changes the human nervous system by affecting memory, behavior, and especially our ability to form social bonds as mammals.

Scientific studies from before 2020 show increased morbidity and mortality due to prolonged isolation. A 2017 study titled "An Overview of Systematic Reviews on the Public Health Consequences of Social Isolation and Loneliness" stated:

> Policy makers and health and local government commissioners should consider social isolation and loneliness as important upstream factors impacting on [sic] morbidity and mortality due to their effects on cardiovascular and mental health. Prevention strategies should therefore be developed.[5]

Several doctors have told me that before the plandemic they were consistently warned by their teachers and supervisors to never isolate patients because of how damaging it is to their mental and physical health.

In 2020, all that sensibility was dismissed.

We were told to stay home and to stand six feet apart in public. Stickers were placed on floors in public places and signs everywhere reminded us of the mandates. Plexiglass barriers were installed at cash registers. People ate at outdoor restaurants with pool noodles attached to hats. People did yoga enclosed in giant plastic balls. People mourning their loved ones were forced to sit far apart at funerals. Children were socially isolated during key developmental periods of their life that depend on social connection.

Devastating elder abuse took place when seniors were isolated from their family members and prohibited from having visitors. They were not allowed to have advocates visit them in hospitals where they underwent medical assault. Many of them died alone. In 2020, a woman at a nursing home was sitting outside in her wheelchair with a sign that read, "I'd rather get COVID than not see my family."

Let us not forget the absolute *insanity* of what happened lest we repeat it in the future.

Just a few years after the forced isolation and social distancing, we are now seeing the downstream effects of the prolonged isolation impairing the ability to form social bonds, even after the isolation period has ended. Children are having difficulty making friends and mental illness is skyrocketing. Adults are more defensive, irritable, and isolated than ever. This is visible on social media, in online forums, on dating apps as well as in real life. We are struggling to truly connect now because our defensive reactions are sabotaging human connection.

The threat of disconnection conditions the nervous system to have hyper-reactive defense responses (fight, flight, freeze, and fawn). This makes it difficult to truly connect because we are triggering each other's defense mechanisms.

When the defense system is activated, the attachment system is offline. The nervous system is binary. It's either in a state of "safe and social" as Dr. Stephen Porges names it in the Polyvagal Theory (a.k.a. rest and digest) or a state of danger, threat, and disconnection.

We have been gaslit about the health consequences of prolonged isolation and loneliness in order to justify the control measures. While these devastating trends are partially being acknowledged now in mainstream media, the acknowledgments are wrapped in the gaslighting of justification that it was necessary to save lives. In other words, they're saying they had to sacrifice our health and wellbeing to protect our health and wellbeing.

There will be long-term consequences for the physical and mental health of individuals and society due to what happened. Perhaps decades from now, with increasing social consciousness, this period in history will be known as The Pandemic of Disconnection.

CHAPTER 2

PARAMETER TWO

Acts of Perceived Kindness

This tactic is meant to build up the target while simultaneously breaking down the target. Acts of perceived kindness are part of an ongoing intermittent reinforcement campaign. The back and forth between sweet and mean, calm and chaos, is the hallmark of the abuse cycle.

Abusers instinctually set up this cycle of intermittent reinforcement, which is what creates cognitive dissonance, brain fog, and confusion. Even though they are cruel and mean, they also intentionally dose the target with acts of perceived kindness.

They have to give you something in order for the abuse and manipulation to work.

Every tyrant uses the same tactic—from the interpersonal to the societal level. Stalin occasionally gave food to the starving masses. While discussing this topic with a man I encountered in a cigar lounge one day, he said he knew someone who used to beat his girlfriend with a wire hanger, then draw her a bath.

It's confusing when the abuser is both the perpetrator *and* the hero. Abusers hurt you and seemingly save you from the very things they did to hurt you. When you call out the abusive things they did, they redirect your attention to their acts of perceived kindness in order to rationalize their "good" character and qualify their intentions.

The goal is for the targets to relax their guard and trust the perpetrators. Eventually the targets will outsource their power to the abusers. This process involves an extortion of trust through seduction—though not necessarily sexual in nature. It can be any kind of verbal flattery, acts of service, gifts, attention, or other gestures that cause a person to feel pleasure, which is a welcome change from the pain.

The acts of perceived kindness can also include temporary reprieves from the abuse that are given from time to time.

It can also involve *future faking*, which is when the manipulator makes false promises of good things that will happen if you continue to show your compliance, loyalty, and good behavior. The target becomes motivated to work harder toward that goal, which is unreachable.

Abusers will tell you things you want to hear, such as calling you a hero for complying, telling you that you're their savior, that they couldn't have done it without you, or even that they can't survive without you. They'll praise you in all sorts of acts of love-bombing. They'll also occasionally reward you in other ways for your compliance and complicity.

Acts of perceived kindness come with strings attached. This parameter creates a distortion around receiving assistance, help, love, and care. The target unknowingly becomes obligated to the unspoken terms and conditions of the abuser's whims. It's a covert contract implying, "You owe me." The abuser will hold these seemingly kind acts over the target's head in order to emotionally manipulate the target's trust.

The acts of perceived kindness are also used as reconnaissance—to extract and gather information about the target's insecurities, fears, desires, and weaknesses, which can later be used for more effective psychological warfare.

Flattery as a weapon

Verbal flattery is one of the most common acts of perceived kindness.

In *Outwitting the Devil*, Napoleon Hill describes his imaginary conversation with the devil in order to understand the tactics used by the dark forces to control humanity: "Flattery is the chief bait with which my agents weave their way into the confidence of people from whom they procure information needed to carry on warfare."[6]

The devil admits to Hill that non-drifters are not easily flattered. Those who are influenced by flattery easily become victims of *the drifting habit*, as Hill named it. When people are drifting, they're easily controllable by the dominant forces in the environment.

> Flattery is a bait of incomparable value to all who wish to gain control over others. It has powerful pulling qualities because *it operates through two of the most common human weaknesses: vanity and egotism*. There is a certain amount of vanity and egotism in everyone. In some people, these qualities are so pronounced they literally serve as a rope by which one may be bound. The best of all ropes is flattery.[7] (Emphasis added.)

People who are easy prey for flattery are captives of their own desires and easily malleable by manipulators.

Perpetrators also aim to lure targets into the unhealthy habits of wrath, envy, pride, sloth, greed, gluttony, and lust in the pursuit of their untamed desires. They'll seduce through flattery, initially rewarding the target for engaging in these distorted desires. That might feel perversely satisfying if we're desperate for permission, attention, validation, approval, pleasure, or power.

Inevitably, the indulgence in disordered desires will consume your soul and distort your perception of self, making you feel unworthy, disgusted, ashamed, lost, and full of regret.

Regrets are like a heavy weight on the heart and soul of a human with a conscience. In fact, this is the part that hurts the most in the aftermath of abuse. The most painful memories are not usually those of what the abuser did, but rather what you did (or didn't do) in reaction to the abuse and how you betrayed yourself.

Perpetrators do this in order to hold those actions over the target's head. The targets start to believe that they are bad and defective, which is what the abusers want them to believe. That shame only gives the abusers more control. So, when they offer flattering words, the target is even more hungry to hear them and lean in.

The perception of kindness

The key is that these acts are *perceived* as kindness. It can be genuine kindness or not. Without energetic discernment, the mind and nervous system can't detect the difference. Sometimes it's so covert at first, that only time can reveal the truth.

When people seem kind, it's natural to want to like them and extend trust to them.

Some abusive relationships start with an intense love-bombing phase where these perceived acts of kindness are introduced. The manipulator will often shower the target with compliments, words of affirmation, gifts, money, dinners, trips, attention, future promises, even physical affection and sex.

Yet while the love-bombing is taking place, there are always subtle signs of the devaluation, meanness, and cruelty mixed in. In most abusive relationships, there's often more building up initially, then more breaking down later. However, in retrospect, people often realize that the intermittent reinforcement of the cycle of abuse was not only a long-term game. It was always taking place during the same day, and sometimes even in the same conversation.

The intermittent reinforcement also causes hormonal conditioning, which affects the dopamine circuit. That's how the alternation of perceived kindness and cruelty induces a motivational state in the target. The target starts to work harder and invest more in the situation in order to get the intermittent rewards.

Many people wonder in retrospect, how did the abuser know which acts of kindness will be most effective? Manipulators will use data mining tactics to gain information about their target during this phase.

In society, we have voluntarily shared much personal information on social media. Our data has also been harvested from those platforms and directly from our devices via covert cyber abuse. That information can be analyzed by supercomputers to be used against us. A supercomputer can do the same type of data analysis, albeit much faster and perhaps more accurately than a human abuser, in order to predict the reaction of a target to certain stimuli. Now with quantum computing, this is exponentializing.

Our data is being used against us to manipulate our emotions, perception, and behavior through messaging campaigns, most of which we are unaware of. Nazi propagandist Joseph Goebbels asserted that propaganda works best when those who are being manipulated are confident they are acting on their own free will.

Cognitive dissonance

Idealization and love-bombing are the tactics used in narcissistic abuse for the purpose of gaining trust and likability. Receiving the intermittent rewards can be addicting, which causes the target to relax his or her guard and dismiss red flags indicating that something is off.

If you're talking with an abuse victim you might notice that in one moment she is telling you how awful her situation is, and, then, the next day or even the next hour, she is idealizing the abuser and talking about all the kind things he does.

When you're observing that from the outside you can almost see something like a short circuit happen in the target's brain. One moment the person is lucid, and in another moment the person is fully in the trance again, unreachable by your voice of reason or the evidence you provide. If you insist on convincing the target that the perpetrator is harming her, she might get angry and even attack you in order to defend the fantasy she wants to believe.

One of the earliest signs of narcissistic abuse is the confusion that a victim feels. Of course, confusion can be caused by other inner conflicts. However, in the case of abusive relationships and situations, the state of confusion is the result of the cognitive dissonance created by the acts of perceived kindness and "good" times mixed with the devaluation, cruelty, and chaos.

Cognitive dissonance is a coping mechanism that makes the brain want to focus on the "good" times or the "good" in the abuser. While that is the innate, intelligent response in childhood so that a kid can survive an intensely stressful and unsafe environment, it becomes maladaptive in adulthood when a person gives his or her power away to an abusive person, group, or situation. The target will become highly motivated to get back to the "good" times, often at a great cost.

In society, people wanted to get "back to normal," as in the pre-2020 world. Of course, if we are really honest, we can admit that things weren't normal before 2020, we were just *normalizing* them.

The stressful inner conflict of cognitive dissonance is between two conflicting and opposing thoughts, beliefs, or perceptions of reality. For example, part of the target knows that something is off and that he is being mistreated. But another part of the target wants to believe that this person is the love of his life, or that his mom or dad really loves him, or that the government actually cares about him and wants to keep him safe.

It sounds something like: "S/he loves me, s/he loves me not…"

A target will often give the benefit of the doubt to the perpetrator through rationalizations. It will sound something like: "S/he didn't mean it that way. S/he did that because s/he cares. S/he really wants the best for me."

Cognitive dissonance keeps an abuse victim in states of denial and defensiveness, not wanting to see the ugly truth and continuing to be loyal to a person who is causing harm. This is what Dr. Patrick Carnes describes as "insane loyalty" in his book *The Betrayal Bond*.[8]

It's the act of perceived kindness that produces the hope that positive change will happen, even while the victim is being destroyed and drained. The seeming kindness becomes an obstacle to choosing health, sanity, freedom, peace of mind, wellness, and personal growth. Making the choice to turn away from the manipulation will require giving up the intermittent rewards and pleasure that are a distraction from the pain.

What is the force so powerful that a person would continue to sacrifice himself in such a situation? It's the dopamine that gets released with the inconsistency of reward. The hope of praise or pleasure is a powerful motivator.

The dopamine evokes a motivational state that causes the target of abuse to work harder for approval and willingly comply with increasingly irrational demands, escalating levels of self-sacrifice and even ridiculously absurd rituals. It's all overlooked for the hope of receiving the reward, the promises of change, or to one day get back to the "good" times.

It's very tempting to stay stuck in the cognitive dissonance. The fantasy, illusion, and toxic hope for a situation that's never going to get better is easier to maintain than the threat of massive disruption that will come with accepting the ugly truth. The latter comes with disillusion, disappointment, devastation, and a very painful abstinence syndrome, which, according to some clients I've worked with, can feel more intense than heroin withdrawal.

In the aftermath of narcissistic abuse (and also during moments of the silent treatment), the target will go through withdrawal, similar to that which drug addicts experience. The only difference is that this drug is endogenous, coming from the body's own chemistry.

Abuse victims can become obsessed with their abusers. But it's not actually the abuser that the person misses. It's the dopamine, how the victims feel when they have the hope of receiving the reward, praise, or pleasure. This trap is especially sticky for people with unresolved childhood trauma where the same dynamics happened with a parent or caretaker. Addictive behavior is usually driven by unmet needs from childhood.

It's easy to get stuck in that addiction, losing self-control, dignity, and the capacity for critical thinking. The further down that path the target goes, the less she'll want to realize how the addiction is poorly affecting her entire life. Like any addict, an abuse target will lie to herself. It's very common to lose everything in these kinds of relationships because the addiction to the high is stronger than the willingness to face the ugly truth.

You may have noticed how some people became obsessed with compliance for the intermittent reward during the COVID era.

First, the government locked us down and separated us through domestic confinement and social distancing measures; then it restored some freedoms and loosened some restrictions—an act of perceived kindness.

The government gave away free "vaccines" as well as incentives to get the shots—followed by boosters. Some states in America offered lotteries with rewards of money, French fries, donuts, and guns. In Las Vegas, if you got vaxxed at certain strip clubs, you could get a free lap dance.

Government stimulus money was given to citizens. Loans were offered to small businesses. Unemployment benefits were offered to "non-essential" workers. Forbearance on home mortgages and student loans were offered.

There were also many promises of safety in the propaganda, such as: *It's for your protection, because we care, to keep you safe, it's safe and effective.*

Giving little doses of truth here and there is also an act of perceived kindness for those of us unaware of the abuse. The little doses of truth trick the brain into the state of hope that we are going back to normal, or back to the good times, because the truth is finally coming out. Yet nothing changes.

An abuser doses the target with little admissions of guilt and even sometimes a *fauxpology*, begging for forgiveness with tears and all. The target gets motivated to keep complying and stoking the false hope that it's getting better. But the next day, or even the next hour, it's like nothing happened.

Anytime a target starts to wake up and set boundaries, tries to leave, or otherwise create distance, the perpetrator will use acts of perceived kindness to pull the target back into the abuse cycle.

In order to continue complying over time, the target must sacrifice her sense of self. The target will increasingly want to be praised for good behavior. She can forget her morals, values, integrity, and what most matters to her in the brain fog of psychological warfare.

The golden child programming

In the narcissistic abuse realm, we talk about the roles of the golden child and scapegoat in an abusive family. This can also apply to a workplace or other social system, including society. These roles are part of the dynamics of an abusive relational matrix. This phenomenon has become even clearer in recent years.

The scapegoat is where the family's (or society's) sins and shame are projected. The scapegoat becomes the focus of the problem, instead of the abuser or the abuse. Those who do evil are always in need of a scapegoat so they can distract attention from accountability for their malevolent actions.

The scapegoat is the one who questions the narrative or fights back, often reacting emotionally and acting out. Then the abuser(s), and their enablers, can point the finger at such behavior as the focus of the problem. The scapegoat is shamed, devalued, punished, ostracized, criticized, or otherwise made to believe that he's defective.

For that reason, some people think it's much better to be the golden child than the scapegoat. But life is not fun for the golden child, either. There are long-term consequences for complying with and enabling abuse and tyranny. These consequences affect not only the individual but also the social system in which the individual exists.

To illustrate this in real life, we can look at the parallels between what happens in the family system and in society. In society, the government is the authority figure like the parents are in a family.

The golden child is the one who bends to the pressure for compliance and is rewarded for being a trophy image that makes the family look good on the outside. The golden child follows the rules and is the example to be followed by others in that social system. Compliance brings temporary relief, but comes with much distress in the long-term.

The golden child will receive love, approval, validation, and acceptance only when it meets the demands of the narcissistic parent(s) or other authority figures. Sometimes compliance isn't rewarded with anything but the temporary absence of abuse. The kid learns to continually adjust to the increasingly absurd rules in order to keep getting intermittent rewards. This same dynamic can continue into adulthood and transfer from one kind of relationship to another.

The narcissistic parent(s) will use triangulation to create a sense of competition between children, setting the bar for getting love and approval through compliance. The one who complies the most (in any given moment) is awarded the status of golden child.

The golden child is an enabler and sometimes also an abuser. The golden child becomes an extension of the narcissistic parent(s) or other authority figure(s). That can lead to carrying out abuse by proxy against the other kids in the family or other people in the social system.

The golden child will get programmed with the belief of being special or exclusive. This can create a sense of entitlement and false confidence in the child's talents, skills, or perception of reality.

The golden child is often the one who says he had an amazing childhood, yet is still in denial about his dysfunctional family system. The same fantasy can happen in a workplace or other social system. Many people discover this upon going to the human resources department at their workplace to report abuse, where they get blamed for what happened and realize they're in some kind of twilight zone.

The golden child gets programmed to default into a state of denial when there is abuse and evil in the environment. This programming can endure into adulthood. While the child may have a more primitive sense of denial about what's happening, the golden child as an adult will develop much more sophisticated methods of denial by rationalizing, intellectualizing, minimizing, and otherwise justifying and normalizing the abuse.

The golden child is programmed to sacrifice his own needs, thoughts, opinions, feelings, and perception of reality when these do not align with those of the abusive parent(s) or authority figure(s). The scapegoat will usually fight against this to some degree.

The golden child learns to avoid rebellion and individuation in order to not betray the expectations of the parent(s), who want the kid to remain infantile and dependent, even into adulthood. Likewise, we live in a society where we are intentionally being infantilized through social engineering so that we are dependent on the system.

Due to the intermittent reinforcement of receiving praise and rewards only when the golden children comply (and even still, not every time), this will become part of their identity. They learn that in order to be considered a "good" person, they must comply, even if it's harmful to themselves or others, or goes against their innate sense of right and wrong.

One of the golden child's main survival mechanisms is people-pleasing behavior (fawning), which often develops into self-sacrifice and codependence. The golden child may learn to satisfy others' needs at the expense of her own. The golden child usually lacks the ability to set boundaries and say no because it will mean a loss of praise, approval, and validation, as well as peace in the relationship or environment. In adulthood the golden child easily falls into similar dynamics.

In some cases, golden children can develop a sense of entitlement and grandiosity in order to avoid the deep sense of insecurity and shame. Sometimes they become manipulative and controlling, using others to meet their needs and disregarding others' right to their own individual identity, opinions, boundaries, perspectives of reality, and needs. This becomes the narcissistic way of self-preservation.

Golden children lose their identity and sense of self in order to meet the expectations of the narcissistic parent(s). They'll become enmeshed and addicted to external validation. This creates a tendency to sacrifice individual identity for the family identity when they're praised by the family for being compliant with the family's ideology and narrative. The same thing happens in society, cults, and other social systems, such as in corporate cultures.

Golden children are taught to measure their self-worth based on accomplishments and praise. Since their self-esteem is derived from others and external factors, they often defer to people pleasing in order to avoid feelings of shame, while yearning for other people to fawn over them.

This form of false self-esteem creates a sense of inferiority, jealousy, and unworthiness that is triggered when other people receive praise for accomplishments or are rewarded for compliance. Golden children may want to be around people who make them feel superior and righteous.

Golden children can become high performers or overachievers, often developing a hypersensitivity to criticism and fear of failure or not being good enough. This can show up even when they do accomplish something.

The narcissistic parent(s) will often praise the kids in one breath and subtly devalue them in the next. The kids learn that it's never enough and they always need to work harder to gain the reward. That creates a deep sense of insecurity and scarcity.

Golden children will develop a terrible fear of not being perfect, which leads to perfectionism. That can create an inability to admit mistakes because it will mean a sense of failure and the death of the false ego they've created in order to feel safe. Golden children will often feel self-directed frustration and anger when they don't measure up to the expectations of others or themselves.

Without self-awareness, confronting the truth and working on self-healing, the childhood programming for the golden child is transferred from the dynamic with the narcissistic parent(s) to other abusive authority figures in adulthood, such as government, partners, friends, and bosses.

The golden child seeks praise and reward, then gets used as an example to coerce compliance and conformity from others who want to get praised and rewarded.

We can see the golden child phenomenon in any tyrannical society, as we saw during the COVID lockdown and "vaccine" campaign:

- When people go along with the abusive expectations, demands, and non-sensical rules of tyrants, even if they disagree or the measures are harmful to them;
- When people compete for the most perfect citizen award and report those who do not comply;
- When people virtue signal their compliance (such as posting about their social distancing actions, wearing masks in selfies, posting photos of their kids in masks, taking *vaxxies* after getting injected);

- When people minimize, rationalize, or otherwise make excuses for the abuse of tyrants who are rewarding them for compliance;
- When people overestimate their own skills or abilities (such as critical thinking) or the righteousness of their compliant actions and participation in abuse of others by proxy;
- When people lose their minds upon being confronted with uncomfortable evidence about the lies and deception coming from government, science, medical systems, academia, corporations, and private organizations because it challenges their ego's image of goodness and perfection for complying, as well as their identity in that system;
- When people pretend that nothing is happening, even when they see the abuse, in order to avoid losing rewards, such as status, privileges, or resources; or
- When people sacrifice reality, reason, facts, or even their life for the praise, flattery, or favor of others.

There was a lot of messaging to promote these behaviors in society. Interestingly, the more educated people are, the more likely they were to believe in and comply with the pandemic measures. Nowadays, academia involves much political indoctrination. Also, the more time, energy, money, and other resources that people invest in getting degrees and status in that system, the less likely they are to see the lies and deception.

Being part of an exclusive group speaks to the golden child programming. That's why celebrities were recruited to influence others by posting their *vaxxies*. Hashtags were used to promote the injections, such as #ImABigShot.

With the goal of "curbing vaccine hesitancy" and "getting more shots in arms" some vax sites were making it easy for people to take and share selfies by setting up a backdrop similar to what one may see at a red carpet event. *Vaxxies* were described as "evidence that selfies can sometimes be selfless."[9] This is classic golden child messaging.

Unfortunately for those who complied, the praise was short-lived, as it is for any golden child. The goal post will always be moved. The bar for praise and approval keeps rising, just like how the golden child will never be enough for the demands of their narcissistic parent(s).

It didn't take long to move the goal post from one shot to two shots to boosters every year. Canada announced that it's no longer using the phrase "fully vaccinated" and instead changed the language to "up to date."[10] Canadians were required to get another dose every nine months in order to get, and maintain, that societal stamp of approval. Some people are still participating in this abuse.

The societal golden child gains a false sense of self-esteem and self-worth from the social praise for compliance. Many people found a new identity in the praise they were getting for being a golden child in society. Social media sites offered stickers to put on avatar photos so that people could virtue signal about getting their shots.

We could all fall into the trap of seeking social approval if we aren't careful to evaluate *why* we do what we do.

Speaking the truth about abuse in an abusive system will always make you a scapegoat of the abusers and their enablers. You can go from being a golden child to a scapegoat in an instant for taking such a stand.

It's far more fun to get praised than punished, devalued, cancelled, and smeared. But that kind of praise comes with a *big* cost that is often overlooked in the moment of instant gratification. Compliance leads to reward in an abusive system, yet it comes with grave consequences.

Over time, only a shell of the original person remains. This is because the person progressively sacrifices his entire identity and sense of self in order to gain the praise (or at least temporarily avoid) the abuse.

In Germany after World War II, most people who had complied with the Nazi tyranny lost their identity. Some of them admitted to their families on their deathbed that they knew what was happening but chose to look the other way. It was easier, and they thought it was safer. So, they pretended things were fine and complied, becoming enablers and accomplices to crimes against humanity.

Pretending damages the heart. The heart is the seat of courage. It takes courage to speak the unpopular truth and risk social rejection. This can feel like a life threat to the mammalian part of our nervous system, which seeks safety through social connection.

The longer we pretend everything is okay when it's not, the more difficult it is to resuscitate courage. Yet the awesome thing is that courage can be contagious, too.

CHAPTER 3

PARAMETER THREE

Perceived Life Threat

Fear is the currency of control in an abusive relationship, family, or society.

The perceived life threat is delivered through a bombardment of fear messaging. The goal is to paralyze the target with an intensely stressful emotional overwhelm. Whether it's a real-life threat or not, what matters is how the nervous system and subconscious mind perceive it. That perception becomes the person's reality.

Many abuse targets fear they will be killed if they try to leave their situation, call out the abuse, or don't comply with what the abuser wants. However, the perceived life threat isn't necessarily limited to the belief that the abuser can, or will, physically end the target's life. The abuser might also threaten the lives of the target's friends or family if the target doesn't cooperate and comply. The abuser could also manufacture an exterior life threat, making the target believe that the only safe space is with the abuser as the protector.

Sometimes perpetrators will manufacture a perceived life threat, and other times they will simply take advantage of one that happens to be occurring. They can be very resourceful and meticulous with this parameter. As con-men and con-women, they're adept at looking for opportunities to exploit to their benefit.

An abuser usually also plays the role of the target's protector or rescuer from such manufactured or real fears, which is an act of perceived kindness, as we explored in Chapter 2. The abuser has already been spinning this narrative—the gaslit version of reality—through information control and isolation, which was the focus of Chapter 1.

The parameters of the state of captivity all layer upon one another to create a bigger picture where it's all connected and leads to the same end goal.

Abusers use fear bombardment and shock trauma tactics, such as reckless driving with the target as a passenger, or coercing the target to do something risky. They could also terrorize the target with other threats like disease, violence, public shaming, war, destituteness, losing children, or anything else that feels life-threatening.

When people start speaking the truth about their family's or partner's abuse, they often have dread attacks, which feel like utter terror. The nervous system usually perceives a life threat when a person reveals these secrets.

Humans are like pack animals in that we are biologically wired to rely on the herd for survival. We can easily forget that nowadays, because of our modern lifestyle.

Character assassination through smear campaigns, rejection, and ostracism could trigger intense fears that feel like a life threat to the nervous system. A person could feel alone in the world or unable to trust her family and close loved ones. Sometimes the perpetrator directly threatens to leave the target or kick her out on the street.

The terror campaign could be much more subtle if a person was already programmed this way since childhood by parents or caretakers. In fact, abusers are often adept at sensing which people would make good targets, even without knowing their life history yet.

In cases of childhood abuse or neglect, the conditioning for the state of captivity happened in early life, so it's much easier to fall into it in adult relationships and situations.

Kids in abusive family systems are helpless, completely dependent on their parents or caretakers for survival. At the time, it's a life threat to be rejected, abandoned, or neglected. For that reason, children in unsafe situations usually learn quickly that fighting for themselves, or speaking the truth, isn't an option.

As adults, the silent treatment, stonewalling, and unexplained disappearances can trigger the same cues of life threat to a person's nervous system. This can be true for humans in general due to our neurological wiring as mammals. The reaction is more amplified for people who experienced the trauma of isolation in childhood.

Every time a perceived life threat happens, that trigger can cause the traumatized target to regress into a childlike state of defenselessness. This state is known as "freeze" or immobilization, which can lead to shut down and collapse.

Freezing is what happens when a mouse is caught in the jaws of a cat. The mouse feigns death as a last-ditch effort to survive. The mouse doesn't make a conscious choice to freeze—it's the autonomic nervous system that takes over. If the mouse is lucky, and a hawk spots the cat, the mouse might have a chance to get loose and mobilize, engaging the flight defense in order to run away.

Freezing is meant to be a very short-term state because the body is feigning death. It's shutting down vital systems, such as respiration, heart rate, and digestion in order to survive.

However, as humans, we can get stuck in long-term, life-threatening situations, such as abuse and tyranny. We can't stay in the freeze state too long because the body is literally dying.

When the fear, shock, and sense of life threat is overwhelmingly stressful, a person can actually die of "vagal death," which Dr. Stephen Porges also refers to as *brachycardyhypoxia*.

The human nervous system usually adapts to ongoing perceived life threats by fleeing from the freeze state into dissociation. That means a person will zone out, disconnect mind and body, turn to substances, or shift into a fantasy world so he doesn't have to feel the emotional or physical pain. For a human, flight doesn't necessarily mean physically fleeing a situation. It can also be fleeing from reality.

The functional freeze state

The term *functional freeze* is a dissociative state that people can get stuck in for days, weeks, months, or years in order to continue surviving a post-traumatic, terrifying or overwhelmingly stressful situation.

In such a state, the person will often be going through the motions, yet losing motivation to take action on anything beyond basic work and life responsibilities. The person is still somewhat functional, so it's not a complete shut down or collapse. It's like running on automaton mode—functioning in a robotic, disconnected, numb, and semi-shutdown way.

Yet despite not doing much, there's an enduring sense of exhaustion for seemingly no reason. It's more than a burnout. This state can continue even after the perceived life threat has ended because the state of captivity is still the program running internally.

A functional freeze state could lead to behaviors like binge-watching TV, videos, series and movies, mindless scrolling on the phone or social media, staring at a page in a book without remembering what you read, losing track of time, frequent bumping into furniture, fixtures, or door frames, feeling aimless and purposeless, easily overwhelmed by small things and procrastinating, canceling or avoiding social situations in general, or showing up but being checked out and unable to truly connect.

This state comes with emotional numbness as well as a background baseline anxiety or depression that the person may or may not recognize because he is so used to it. Hypervigilance is common, as well as the mental paralysis caused by indecision or fear. There's a disconnection from self, others, and *All That Is*.

In the functional freeze state, people often gain weight, even if they're exercising and eating healthily. This is because the metabolism is affected. Alternatively, some people might not feel hungry or forget to eat, so they might lose weight.

Even though the functional freeze is more like the flight response of dissociation, the person will frequently get triggered into the full-on freeze state. While each of those triggers is usually of short duration, it's extremely draining of energy.

When perceived life threats trigger the nervous system into collapse and shutdown, it becomes more severe. That's when people often can't function enough to hold down a job or even meet their basic hygiene needs. This state is very common for those with post-traumatic stress. Taking a shower and brushing teeth can feel like monumental activities when a person has no energy or drive to live.

Getting sick more often is common because the immune system is also down when we are in a freeze state. Many clients I've worked with who were in abusive relationships and situations for decades in childhood or adulthood, or both, ended up with auto-immune issues due to the constant threat of attack in their environment and how their body reacted to those threats.

From a holistic perspective, the immune system represents our boundaries and defenses against invasion or being taken advantage of. It also differentiates self from the other. All that is distorted in abusive relationships and situations.

When a person feels under continual attack, afraid of confrontation, unsure of his right to set boundaries, and often blaming himself for being dysfunctional in order to feel some sense of control over his life, these kinds of dynamics can cause health issues. The more a person struggles with health problems, the deeper he can get stuck in a functional freeze state due to the despair caused by life-altering symptoms. It becomes a vicious cycle.

It's no surprise that so many people are talking about the functional freeze state nowadays in the aftermath of the COVID measures and the state of captivity that was induced in much of the world. However, there seems to be a heightened prevalence of this awareness among Generation Z.

Most of Gen Z is living a 24/7 existence in the virtual world, especially social media. It's easy for someone my age in Generation X to forget that those in Gen Z were born in a time when the digital world was already overlaid on the reality in which they grew up. As Gen Xers, we remember what life was like before the internet, smart devices, and social media. For members of Gen Z, the virtual world can feel more real than the real world because it's all they've known.

The functional freeze trend was starting before the 2020s. The Digital Age was already creating the perfect terrain for it. We have drifted into the habit of co-regulating with technological devices instead of self-regulating and co-regulating with other humans. Many have become dependent on social media for external validation. Online bullying, social judgment, and comparison along with the threat of ostracism can be overwhelming and debilitating, especially to those who already have a history of relational trauma.

The 24/7 digital stress on the nervous system got much worse after youngsters were terrified through the COVID fear campaign and deprived of social contact during key years of their developmental processes and emergence into adulthood.

That may be the main reason why so many in their generation are feeling detached and disengaged from life, goals, relationships, and a sense of purpose in the post-pandemic era. It's not helpful when older generations look down on them and shame them for being "lazy" or feeling stuck in this state. They first need compassion for what happened to them and an understanding of why they adapted in that way so that they can start to shift into empowerment and return to life.

If left unresolved, this ongoing trend will have devastating impacts on the future of humanity because the unresolved trauma and sense of disconnection from life and relationships will get passed down to the kids of Gen Z.

A baby who doesn't receive a healthy emotional attachment through the eye gaze and attuned connection with the mother in the early days, weeks, and months of life will be programmed into a default state of emotional insecurity and relational dysfunction.

A couple years ago, a pregnant woman told me she was planning the nursery for her baby and asking new moms for advice. The number one recommendation they gave her was to have an electrical outlet next to the nursing chair so she could charge her cellphone.

One of my clients from Eastern Europe described the infant of a mother who is looking at her phone instead of in the baby's eyes as a "dead mother" because there's no emotional connection. The autonomic nervous system reads the disconnection as a life threat.

Due to the increasing unresolved trauma and smartphone usage, how many babies nowadays are getting a healthy emotional attachment vs. the imprint of feeling alone and untethered to anything or anyone else?

Why aren't more studies being done on the impact of human co-regulation with digital devices in terms of how it changes our nervous system and ability to connect with each other?

The brain fog of warfare

The freeze and functional freeze states lead to dissociation, which is a flight response accompanied by a heavy brain fog. It becomes hard to think and focus at all when there are frequent life threat triggers. It's very challenging to concentrate and remember things, which leads to all kinds of other problems in relationships, at work, and in life in general.

In the freeze state, people are closed off to new information that could help them to understand and escape their predicament, whether they're still in an abusive situation, or it's over but they're still stuck in the state of captivity.

This is why if you've ever tried to wake up victims of abuse, they usually refuse to see the evidence. In a freeze or dissociation state, people often won't even get angry as they do when they're in the cognitive dissonance that we explored in Chapter 2.

Anger corresponds to a mobilization state in the nervous system. In a freeze state, a person is mostly emotionally numb, exhausted, and immobilized. Maybe you've noticed it when you tried to present information to someone in this state. Her gaze might go blank and she might not even hear or remember what you said.

The freeze state is the lowest state of human consciousness: We are locked out of higher faculties, such as creativity, insight, intuition, critical thinking, and imagination—the inner resources that can help us to figure out how to escape our unhealthy predicament and dissolve our state of captivity.

When the emotional pain and stress of the fear and life threat is severe, endogenous opioids are released to induce a sense of numbness.

That has a survival purpose so we can keep going despite the pain. However, it becomes very difficult to leave an abusive relationship or situation when we are so numb that we can't even feel our circumstances or get angry about it in order to set boundaries and mobilize out of there.

Of course, these survival mechanisms serve the purpose of helping us feel to safe in unsafe environments and situations. During childhood, the freeze response was an innate, intelligent response to survive when we had no other option.

However, these survival mechanisms become maladaptive over the long-term into adulthood, keeping us stuck instead of setting boundaries, mobilizing, and taking action, in order to heal and move forward in life.

Even when people do leave abusive relationships and situations, they're often stuck in a state of inertia indefinitely. It's all so overwhelming that it's easier to shut down or go into the functional freeze state.

If you've been in that state, you know how exhausting it is, which makes it highly challenging to summon the energy needed to overcome the gravitational pull of the fear collapse. In that state, it's so much easier to drift into negativity and settle for unhealthy relationships and situations, including tyranny.

When a person is unable to mobilize out of the state caused by an ongoing perceived life threat, he will start to believe that he is worthless and incapable. Being treated as unworthy and incapable becomes the new normal, often causing a person to start to give up. A person could end up believing that he is not worthy of existing or even having the most basic human rights. Unfortunately, many people are programmed with such beliefs in childhood.

That makes it easy for abusers to get their targets to co-sign on the degradation of their own dignity. Most of this happens unknowingly and by default because the target is immobilized and lacks the clarity of perspective as well as the life force energy to get out of that state. The more you get used to dehumanizing treatment, the more you believe the lie of unworthiness.

Fear as a formidable weapon

Fear is the glue of the trauma bond. In other words, it's at the core of what holds a person in the state of captivity, even after leaving the treacherous person, environment, or situation.

Fear drains a person's life force energy. It collapses the human energy field. It makes us weak and immobile. It lowers immunity.

You would think that public health officials would have been extra careful not to use fear bombardment during a *pandemic*, but they did the exact opposite. They poured fear on an uncertain situation like fuel on a fire.

In 2020, the intense fear bombardment began. The news was constantly pumping fear-based messaging and imagery with a case count and death count on the TV screen every day. Social media platforms were promoting the fear and couching their censorship as a necessary evil against life-threatening information that could spread the virus and kill others.

In 2021, when the medical experiment began, in order to get people to take the shots, many governments, employers, institutions, and businesses coerced people to get vaxxed under the threat of losing their jobs and livelihood, their right to get an education, and their ability to travel or participate in society, such as entering restaurants, cafes, bars, concerts, theaters, sporting events, music festivals, gyms, or even public restrooms.

In America, on September 9, 2021, President Joe Biden issued an executive order requiring all federal employees and contractors, including the military, to get vaxxed. He also forced private companies of one hundred or more employees to coerce their employees to get vaxxed or face fines. It was an unconstitutional mandate, which gave permission to many state-level officials to do the same.

Biden continually called the unvaxxed a threat to public health. He devalued and smeared the minority of people who didn't take the shots, saying, "Twenty-five percent can do a lot of damage, and they are." In the same speech, he went on to push more misinformation: "The unvaccinated overcrowd our hospitals, are overrunning the emergency rooms and intensive care units, leaving no room for someone with a heart attack, or pancreatitis, or cancer."[11]

The *pandemic of the unvaccinated* lie was later revealed to be the opposite of reality. But due to the psychological torture of fear, the brain fog, plus the censorship and information control, most people were too exhausted to do their own research. Instead, they repeated the unsubstantiated narrative of the so-called trusted sources.

President Biden punctuated his threatening message to the unvaxxed: "Our patience is wearing thin."[12] He also threatened: "It will be a winter of severe illness and death for the unvaccinated"[13]—yet it was not.

Weaponized fear corrupts the human operating system, as I wrote in my contribution to *Canary in a Post-Covid World Vol.2: Money, Fear and Power*, a collection of essays from thirty-seven contemporary thought leaders:

> When we look back at what happened since 2020, it's important to start with the question: Who or what was powerful enough to shut down the entire world?
>
> Was it the federal or local governments? The WHO [World Health Organization]? The WEF [World Economic Forum]? The NHS [Britain's National Health Service] or NIH [U.S. National Institutes of Health]? The corporations? The media? The coronavirus?
>
> It was actually none of the above.
>
> If we look at the bigger picture, it was fear that shut down the world.
>
> It was fear that drove billions of people to stay home and choose not to see their loved ones for months or years.
>
> It was fear that caused people to comply with increasingly insane rules created by hypocritical public figures

who were often caught disregarding those very same rules.

It was fear that drove people to roll up their sleeves and participate in a medical experiment—either voluntarily because they feared sickness and death for themselves and others, or involuntarily by coercion or force because they feared losing their jobs, educational opportunities, seeing loved ones, enjoying events, concerts, restaurants, traveling or otherwise participating in society.

It was fear that blinded people from seeing the manipulation and deception in the propaganda.

It was fear that drove people to hate one another.

Biological fear is a natural survival mechanism built into the nervous system. When fear alerts us of a threat in the environment, the defense system automatically gets activated so we can fight or flee from the danger.

However, fear can become a formidable weapon when it's used to manipulate a person's perception and drive their behavior.[14]

The science of fear and compliance

Scientific studies conducted before and during 2020 clearly show how fear and isolation can be used to influence perception and behavior.

The fear mongers sure did *follow the science.*

The fear and isolation tactics deployed to sell all things COVID to the public are the same ones that will be used against us in ongoing manipulation campaigns about the climate, war, economy, food, energy, elections, digital surveillance, designer gene manipulation technology, and other things we can't even imagine yet.

Fear appeals are effective for persuasion, according to the 2015 study "Appealing to Fear: A Meta-Analysis of Fear Appeal Effectiveness and Theories."[15]

This study concluded the following, paraphrased here in plain language:

1. Appealing to fear is effective for influencing attitude, intentions, and behavior.
2. There are very few circumstances in which fear appeals aren't effective.
3. There are no circumstances in which fear appeals backfire and lead to "undesirable" outcomes (for those who spread the fear).
4. Efficacy statements increase the effectiveness of the fear appeals.

In other words, fear can be used to modify perception and behavior. This was part of the basis for the marketing slogan *safe and effective*. People were terrified of death. The use of the word "effective" increased the success of the fear-based messages in getting people to take the experimental injections.

"Safe" is a carrot of hope dangled as promised relief from the relentless fear bombardment, an act of perceived kindness, as we explored in Chapter 2.

The science showed that it's important to dose the masses with hope amidst the fear messaging. A 2019 study, "Uplifting Fear Appeals: Considering the Role of Hope in Fear-Based Persuasive Messages,"[16] discovered that an element of hope can be introduced to increase the success of the fear appeals used to coerce people into certain behaviors.

As mentioned in Chapter 2, the dosing of hope is a tactic employed by all psychological manipulators to numb the target's critical mind, gain compliance, and keep the target in the abuse cycle based on promises for the future.

Hope was the emotional tone of Google's marketing campaign *Get back to what you love*[17]—the same slogan used in YouTube's Vaccine Confidence Project.[18] *The Economist* cover of November 14, 2020, "Suddenly, hope,"[19] was a powerful message for the launch of the jab.

After the relentless fear bombardment, many were desperate to get back to the people, events, and activities that they love and missed. The injections were positioned as the one hope and only escape from that nightmare.

After COVID began and before the vax was unleashed on the public, an interesting study explored using people as pawns to spread the fear, in order to encourage vax uptake. It was called "COVID-19 Vaccine Messaging, Part 1."[20]

In 2020, Yale University studied ten different messages for their effectiveness in selling the jab to the public. These fear-based messages appealed to personal freedom, economic freedom, self-interest, community interest, economic benefit, guilt, embarrassment, anger, trust in science, and bravery.

The study states five primary and secondary outcome measures, their objectives, paraphrased here in plain language:

1. Get people to get vaxxed.
2. Get people to trust the vax.
3. Get people to get other people to get vaxxed.
4. Get people to fear those who are unvaxxed.
5. Get people to socially judge the unvaxxed based on the following parameters: trustworthiness, selfishness, likeableness, and competence.

These fear-based messages were deployed by the media, corporations, organizations, politicians, "philanthropaths,"[21] and influencers, then spread by the masses across social media and society.

An abuser would be powerless without enablers. It's the enablers who maintain an abusive system. This is why the perpetrators had to get the people to do their bidding for them. The same thing happens in every abusive family, workplace, or other social system.

You can replace the vax in the objectives above with any other behavior that an abuser would want the target to comply with, then notice how these tactics are similar to the ones that abusers instinctively use in interpersonal relationships, family systems, workplaces, cults, and other social groups.

Some messages were clearly more effective than others. Those became the standard talking points of the COVID narrative as well as the knee-jerk reactions to anyone questioning the narrative.

Community interest was used in messages like "We're all in this together" and "Do your part."

Trust in science appeared in slogans like "Follow the science," which was combined with embarrassment in *ad hominem* attacks, such as "You're anti-science."

Guilt was the emotional manipulation in curses, such as "You're going to kill grandma."

What was the life threat during all things COVID? Most people were conditioned to fear death by the virus and other people as the vectors of the virus. Other people were afraid of the medical and social tyranny, smear campaigns, ostracism, losing access to healthcare benefits, not being permitted to see loved ones or go to school, losing the ability to earn a living, or the right to move around and travel.

After 2020, we all have a new relationship with fear. How has your relationship with fear changed since then?

Have you done any research on alternative narratives to virology? Is it possible that we've been misled into the fear of contagion when that's not what's actually making people sick?

If you've been in an abusive relationship or other situation, are you now starting to see common patterns between your personal experiences and what happened in society during the COVID campaign?

CHAPTER 4

PARAMETER FOUR

Perceived Inability to Escape

The key to this parameter is that the target feels trapped and doesn't see a way out, even if he or she is allowed to move around freely. Resisting the abuse is painful, so it's easier to comply. However, the abuse keeps escalating and it gets increasingly more difficult to leave.

In the process of abuse programming, the target develops a dependence on the perpetrator for survival. A perceived inability to escape means that people start to believe they can't leave or survive on their own. They become so exhausted and helpless that they don't even try to fight or escape. It feels like it's impossible to leave or stop the abuse and pain, so they surrender to it.

A clear example of this is a woman who experiences marital rape. She learns that if she fights her husband, it will only prolong the inevitable pain. So, she decides to *just let him get it over with*. Likewise, I heard several people say they went to get jabbed *just to get it over with*.

Overt abusers will say things like "You can't leave, how will you make it on your own out there?" Or they'll convince the target, "No one else will love you and put up with you like I do."

In other cases, the abusers might more covertly imply that the target can't leave or survive without them. The covert perpetrators who play the victim will use guilt-tripping tactics, implying that if the target leaves, the abuser will be destroyed and perhaps even die or commit suicide. The targets believe that it would be their fault, and they already feel bad about themselves, so they keep staying.

The covert perpetrator who plays the hero will use superiority messaging to appeal to the target's ego, making the target feel like a good person by continuing to invest in the abusive situation, by default implying that the target would otherwise be a bad person. This corresponds to the golden child programming we explored in Chapter 2.

Perpetrators always test their targets early on in the relationship, friendship, or job to see how accommodating they are, how willing they are to self-sacrifice, and how insecure they are upon hearing or seeing signs of disapproval or disagreement.

The abuse conditioning goes on over time with escalating demands and continual goal-post moving. The target is already motivated to keep investing due to the intermittent reinforcement and dopamine circuit, and eventually it feels like there's no way out.

The goal-post moving could involve future promises of whatever the target most wants, such as a house or living situation, a vacation, an investment, a job, leaving a job, having a child, or even peace from the chaos. There's always some kind of empty promise that keeps the target making these ongoing sacrifices thinking that, one day, it will finally be worth it, so there's no sense in trying to escape.

It's about conditioning the target to accept that there's always something more she needs to do or sacrifice in order to escape the suffering. The pain becomes inescapable.

After so many sacrifices and moving of the goal posts without ever reaching the promised land, the target starts talking herself out of taking any action to change her circumstances, no matter how miserable she is.

By that point she's invested so much, that walking away without any wins feels like an unbearable loss. And deep down, she often doesn't believe that she is worthy or capable of surviving on her own anyway.

Learned helplessness sets in

When a person is psychologically isolated, terrified, and feels like there's no escape, that induces a state of learned helplessness. This results in a sense of debility, dependence, dread, powerlessness, hopelessness, and apathy. In such a state, the person feels that he has no control over his life and nothing he does is enough.

The target's mind eventually gets stuck in the perspective of *I can't.* Perhaps you can relate to this kind of thinking. It sounds something like this:

"I can't leave."

"I can't get divorced, I have kids and property."

"I can't make it on my own out in the world."

"I can't say no."

"I can't survive without…"

"I can't afford to lose…"

"I can't provide for my kids on my own."

After some time in the state of learned helplessness, existential exhaustion and despair set in, leading to spiritual bankruptcy. If you've experienced this, you might relate to feeling like you lost all faith in yourself, others, God, and the possibility of a different way of life.

When all faith is lost, the only thing left is emptiness. This state causes a complete disconnection from self, others and All That Is. This is quite possibly the most painful state a human being can know.

The inability to escape an ongoing and intensely stressful situation will cause a person to engage in fawning behaviors (appeasement), such as caretaking the abusive person, people pleasing, accommodating, and self-sacrificing to the point of self-abandonment.

During a traumatic childhood, a kid might learn to fawn in order to create a sense of safety and avoid conflict in an unsafe environment with unsafe people. This is the intelligent response for a child who has no way out of that situation. However, in adulthood it becomes maladaptive.

Compliance will never end the abuse—it only prolongs it, leading to more destruction and self-destruction. But the survival brain doesn't understand this and is merely trying to keep the person alive through fawning and appeasement behaviors when the person sees no way out. Ongoing compliance leads to escalating abuse, tyranny, and traumatization.

The origins of the fawning response

The fawning response is motivated by intense fear and the perceived inability to escape the circumstances. This sets people up for an adulthood of accommodating and compliance, saying yes when they want to say no, agreeing when they disagree, or self-sacrificing in order to put someone else's needs and feelings first.

They learn to put on a mask to match other people's expectations. That means disregarding their own needs and wellbeing, which leads to emotional imbalance as well as chronic physical and mental illness. Yet none of this behavior is conscious. It's all in the subconscious programming caused by the abuse conditioning.

In childhood, this may have been the only way to get some needs met or at least to avoid being punished, rejected, abandoned, or ignored. Children are helpless and dependent on adults to take care of them and meet their needs. Children can learn to fawn in order to gain safety and acceptance when they only receive approval and love upon doing what they're told.

When the developmental process gets distorted or sabotaged by irresponsible, immature, abusive, or neglectful parents, that sets up children for a challenging adulthood in which they often learn to survive by self-abandoning. Their programming leads to accommodating others in unhealthy ways. They will have a deep craving for external validation in order to feel safe, so they'll put others' needs, feelings, and opinions above their own. In the process they'll develop low self-worth and self-esteem.

If this happened to you in childhood, you might relate to experiences in adulthood where you abandoned your own needs to appease others and avoid conflict. You probably have a hard time saying no for fear of rejection and because you want to keep the peace, making others comfortable or happy.

This programming causes a people to take responsibility for what doesn't belong to them, while not taking responsibility for their own needs, emotions, feelings, and desires.

People-pleasing behavior is different from generosity driven by self-expression. According to *Psychology Today*:

> Children raised by unhealthy parents are often trained to please their parents above pursuing their own interests and proclivities. Significantly impaired parents, such as those suffering from symptoms of borderline personality disorder (BPD), narcissistic personality disorder (NPD), and other serious mental illnesses, often traumatize their children if they do not do what they want. This often occurs through parents lashing out at their children when they are not pleased. These children grow up to be adults who consistently put the well-being of others ahead of their own. They do not do this out of generosity. Instead, they do this to feel safe.[22]

After this kind of childhood trauma, in adulthood you can become hypersensitive to criticism and disapproval. That can cause you to agree to do things, or have things done to you, that you're not okay with because you're afraid to set boundaries. If this is relatable, in childhood you probably learned that you had no right to set boundaries or that it was selfish.

You might have learned to be compliant and helpful in order to prove your worthiness, even when it goes against your values or otherwise harms you in some way. Being helpful was part of your childhood programming to get your needs met or to avoid abuse. In adult relationships, you're likely to stay in toxic relationships beyond the expiration date, continually trying to prove you're good enough and afraid to say no.

Abusers and manipulators are very drawn to the fawning types because they are ideal prey. They want a target who will continue to accommodate, going along to get along. Abusers love compliance because it makes them feel powerful and significant.

The COVID campaign was all about compliance and most of the world fawned to some degree, going along for the ride in order to avoid the conflict, rejection, and punishment. Understandably, saying no and setting boundaries came with a cost, but so did complying. It felt like there was no way out.

Sometimes a relationship or situation reaches a breaking point, where the target wakes up and realizes he wants out because he can't keep living like that. In order to do so, he must overcome the gravitational pull of the inertia and learned helplessness. It can feel so daunting that a person doesn't see a way out and continues to stay despite the awareness of how unhealthy it is.

One of the biggest challenges to leaving an abusive relationship or situation is to accept that the person, corporation, government, or whatever it may be, doesn't actually love you or want the best for you. The acts of perceived kindness make it confusing and all too easy to justify that *they really do love you in their own way*. It's not surprising that so many people blindly trust governments and corporations. They learned this at home.

The abuse cycle feels inescapable

Once you get into the abuse cycle, it's challenging to get out, but not impossible. Of course, it's better to get out before the devil shows his horns. However, most people get pulled in unknowingly by giving the benefit of the doubt, which logically sounds like the reasonable and kind thing to do.

It's not easy to accept that evil exists in this world. That's one of the biggest obstacles we face when it comes to liberating ourselves from the state of captivity.

Many people are currently in the process of learning these painful lessons in their relationships and life. Since we are all connected in the abusive system of society, we are going to feel the pain in one way or another, though we can certainly opt out as much as possible. It's also painful to watch loved ones (or even strangers) fall into the abuse cycle and suffer as narrative after narrative gets spun to trap people into it. For example, some people escaped the COVID campaign, then immediately fell into the war propaganda.

In February 2022, almost overnight, many people changed their online avatar photo stickers from their vax virtue signal to the Ukraine flag. In Texas, where I was living at the time, the state flag is sacred. Many businesses fly the Texas flag and the American flag together. It was shocking to see how quickly the Texas flag was replaced with the Ukraine flag as I drove down the highway through Dallas.

The fog of any war is always thick with propaganda. As the war themes continue to escalate, each time the government and media bombard us with fear of the declared enemy and inform us of the narrative we must adopt to maintain golden child status, lest they smear us as conspiracy theorists, racists, or other derogatory terms. Celebrities and other influencers are recruited to set the example of the golden child in society to be followed. Once you see the pattern, you can't unsee it.

The perpetrators will continue to manufacture fear scenarios while making promises that they're going to fix things. They just need you to do something for them—whether to vote for them, to stop traveling, to stop eating meat or eggs, to stay home and socially distance, to take pharmaceuticals, to give up your human rights and dignity, to consent to the digital surveillance grid in the name of security, or to plug yourself into biotechnology *for the greater good.*

The abuse cycle causes people to beg their abusers for a solution or justice. That's when the abusers offer their pre-meditated solution that they wanted to drive us toward all along. I hope that by now you're noticing the same patterns repeat themselves in all kinds of issues in the news. It's the Hegelian dialect of Problem–Reaction–Solution. The same happens in interpersonal relationships, families, and workplaces.

Abusers create a problem or take advantage of one already occurring. They stoke your emotional reaction through gaslighting and fear bombardment, getting you to demand something be done. They entice you to outsource your power to them through acts of perceived kindness and empty promises. Then you start to believe that they have the solution that can save you from these circumstances, so you give up your personal sovereignty (and sometimes much more) for a rescue fantasy. That's how you can end up accepting the solution they wanted to provide all along while maintaining yourself in a state of captivity.

Escapism as a coping mechanism

When a person believes that he can't escape the abusive relationship or otherwise intensely stressful situation, he will turn to escapism behaviors and distractions, such as food, drinking, drugs, porn, sex, gambling, shopping, movies and series, social media scrolling, or workaholism. Rescue fantasies are another form of escapism.

The trauma of the abuse programming installs a spiritual parasite that causes the person to feel intense self-destructive impulses. Escapism leads to self-destruction through unhealthy habits. In severe cases, the escapism can reach extreme levels leading to self-harm and suicide.

Sometimes chronic illness and a health crisis wake people up and motivate them to get out. Some people are fortunate enough to have a holistic-minded doctor who asks the right questions and sees the connection between the trauma in the person's life and the body's response. Sometimes people also have that awakening by divine grace when they realize their body cannot go on like that and they finally have the motivation to choose a new path.

For others, the only escape is death because their soul doesn't see another way out. Many domestic abuse victims never get out and instead take their situation to the grave with illness or suicide.

In October 2024, Canada's death review panel approved and euthanized the first person who chose to be put out of his misery by Medical Assistance in Dying (MAiD) due to a vax injury named "controversial post COVID-19 vaccination syndrome."[23]

Is the recent global increase in euthanasia programs another socially engineered escapism option for population control? Or is it because the social engineers care and want the best for us?

Escapism caused by the COVID campaign

The entire COVID psychological operation was set up so that the only escape and way out from the fear, intense stress, and loss of normality was the vaccine that was promised to save us all.

In the early 2020s, most people were conditioned to believe there was no escape from the COVID fear and life threat as well as everything they had to give up along the way. This stopped people from thinking critically and investigating if the danger was as serious as we were being told.

As we explored in the first few chapters, when we are confused with cognitive dissonance, paralyzed by fear, and feel trapped in the immobilization, that's often when it's the most challenging to investigate and think clearly. Most of the world bought into the fear to some degree because of the intensity of the fear bombardment, the acts of perceived kindness, and our inability to let our higher human consciousness see another perspective.

Because people didn't see a way out of the neurological, psychological, and spiritual torment, escapism behaviors, such as drinking, soared in 2020. Porn use increased as well. Many people retreated into fantasy because it was easier than facing reality. Drug use increased and overdoses soared. Many turned to substances to give themselves a sense of control and escape.

During the lockdowns in 2020, some doctors said that they saw more suicides in a month than they normally see in a year.

During the COVID fear campaign, the goal posts kept moving. First it was two weeks to slow the spread, then it became a month, then several months. We were told that we had to wear masks in public. If you didn't want to cover your breathing holes, enablers would say, "It's just a mask." It was easier to comply than to keep fighting.

Those of us who were watching the incremental escalation of mandates knew that it wasn't going to stop at the mask. Sure enough, the goal post moved to the shot. Then, it was two shots. Then a booster. And another booster. By then most people stopped complying, but that's only because it wasn't forced or coerced any more.

After the Canadian trucker protest gained traction in early 2022, the global narrative quickly pivoted to the war in Ukraine as if the prior two years never happened.

Following the biggest psychopathic con in the history of humanity, it was incredibly bizarre how the COVID campaign was suddenly dropped with no explanation or closure. Other than some lingering reminders in the media and by corporations like drug stores and grocery stores to keep getting boosted, it was like we were left to pretend that nothing had happened as new narratives, such as war and energy scarcity, were moved into the headlines.

This created a surreal sensation and unresolved trauma that we were expected to just forget and move on without closure. But trauma isn't healed by forgetting. There is no moving forward until we resolve the past. The state of captivity doesn't go away on its own.

The abuse always escalates

People often ask abuse survivors why they didn't leave or why they didn't see the abuse. It's very difficult to see when you're in it. It's like being in a hypnotic trance. Once people realize and get out of the relationship or situation, it's often shocking for them to look back and realize what they tolerated.

Abuse and degradation escalate over time. It's important to understand that *abuse doesn't start where it ends.*

It starts slowly, with gradual increments over time to avoid setting off internal alarm bells. Every time a person goes through that abuse cycle in a relationship, things intensify. The abuse escalates. The victim's tolerance to the abuse also escalates. In that process, it's easy to forget who you are. You might even forget that you are worthy of basic human dignity.

Hindsight is 2020. Maybe that's going to be the morbid cosmic joke some years or decades down the road. After people have seen the downstream effects of those measures, perhaps they'll ask, *how could such a thing have happened?*

There's a predictable pattern of abusive behavior in interpersonal relationships, just as there is for abusive behavior by tyrants within a society.

If an abuse victim tries to tell others what's happening before the signs are overt, it's likely that people won't believe the victim. Instead, they'll say things like "I'm sure s/he loves you and wants the best for you" or "You're reading too much into that."

These are similar to the minimization catch phrases that people use in society, such as what happened during the COVID campaign: "Public health officials care about saving lives," and "you're being paranoid, this is about the health of everybody."

Now we have an excessive amount of people dying suddenly and others developing all kinds of physical, psychological, and spiritual health crises due to the long-term effects of the medical and social experiments that took place. We've only begun to see the cumulative consequences of what was done in the recent years. As writer Margaret Anna Alice poignantly outlined, "Mistakes Were NOT Made."[24]

The distorted pursuit of peace vs. non-compliance

Most of us want to live in peace. However, there are circumstances in which the desire for peace can become toxic. This is what happens for people who were programmed since childhood to be a peacemaker in the family. It's very common for those who grew up in dysfunctional families with abuse, neglect, addictions, spiritual bypassing, toxic positivity, and other unhealthy dynamics.

That conditioning causes the child to sacrifice her own needs, feelings, and wellbeing in order to feel safe. This is done by maintaining the peace through compliance and caretaking of the authority figures. The trauma programming carries into adulthood, leading to codependence and self-sacrifice in relationships, and a further loss of self.

But there's another choice. It's easy to forget this option once you're all in. The only end to the insanity of doing the same thing and expecting different results is to opt out of the game—to stop complying.

Why do people comply with abuse and tyranny? They get temporary relief from the gnawing anxiety and fear.

Imagine you don't want to talk to someone, but that person keeps calling and texting incessantly. Every time you see another call or text, your anxiety level rises. Your instinct might be to answer the phone or send a text to get the person to stop, which will temporarily relieve your anxiety. But it's going to keep happening.

Likewise, complying with abuse will not lead to your freedom. Ask anyone who did what the school bullies wanted. It only gets worse. It's never enough to fill an abuser's insatiable desire for control.

Every time you do what abusers tell you to do, you're teaching them what you'll accept and do, so naturally they're going to do more of it. Abusers in relationships, families, workplaces, communities, and societies will keep moving the goal post as long as people keep playing along. Abusers keep taking. Enablers keep normalizing and complying. The abusers can only get away with it if they have participants in that game.

Where will you draw the line and say *enough*?

That evil game only works with our participation. We can either maintain the abusive system by complying with the role written for us, or we can opt out. It's not an easy decision, and both options come with risks as well as losses, but only one of these paths leads to any real and lasting empowerment, liberation, and inner peace.

This is where our responsibility comes in. We are not responsible for what other people do. Our power is in our choices and how we respond to other people and life. When we make new choices, we get new results.

Ending the compliance will come with temporary pain in the short term in order to gain peace in the long run. One of the most important life lessons I've learned is *don't sacrifice your long-term peace for peace in the moment.*

CHAPTER 5

STATE OF CAPTIVITY

The Locus of Control Is Within

The four parameters we explored induce a state of captivity. This state of consciousness alters a person's perspective and behavioral response to life. That kind of conditioning tricks us into outsourcing our power to someone or something external.

The progression into this state is not a linear process. All four parameters are layered and stacked like octaves, simultaneously building on the psychological, neurological, and spiritual state of captivity.

It is an escalating cycle of love-bombing and devaluation involving the core four elements: isolation, acts of perceived kindness, perceived life threats via fear bombardment, and the perception that there's no way out.

The cycling nature of these relationships and situations continually pressures the target into thinking that her only option is compliance. That's how the target becomes an emotional, mental, and spiritual hostage. This is why physical confinement isn't necessary.

The predicament of traumatic entrapment and the oppression of darkness is not resolved by simply leaving and allowing time to pass. Unfortunately, time itself does not do the healing.

The unresolved trauma keeps a person in a state of defense (fight, flight, freeze, and fawn). When we are on defense, we aren't on offense. That means we are reacting to others and life instead of being pro-active and creating the life that we want to live. It feels like someone or something else is in control.

It also means being locked in lower states of consciousness, without access to our higher faculties of human consciousness like critical thinking, creativity, imagination, insight, and intuition. We become increasingly more disconnected from self, others, and God, the Creator of All That Is, Spirit, Source, infinite intelligence, or whatever you call your higher power.

Psychological abuse is spiritual warfare. It's uncanny that abusers instinctually know how to lure in their prey and keep their victims stuck in the abuse cycle. Regardless of gender, country, culture, language, socioeconomic status, and ethnicity, the patterns of psychological abuse are the same.

The only possible explanation for this phenomenon is spiritual. *They're all serving the same master.* It's the same energetic force of darkness behind it all. That force of evil and negativity goes by many names. I expose the darkness more in Chapter 10.

In *Wild at Heart*, John Eldredge explains his perspective of spiritual warfare and how the Evil One comes between us. The same principles can be applied to the macro level in society.

First, the Adversary takes out comms.

Eldredge writes, "Before an effective military strike can be made, you must take out the opposing army's line of communication. The Evil One does this all the time—in ministries and especially with couples."[25] He emphasizes the importance of prayer and connection with God to counteract the distorting messages we may receive. "Most of all the Enemy will try to jam communications with Headquarters."[26]

This fits with the first parameter of the state of captivity: isolation. In Chapter 1, I described how the isolation is physical and psychological. I explained how abusers control and manipulate the information in relationships, families, workplaces, and social groups as well as in society. This also happens in our relationship with our higher power.

The distorted information makes it difficult for people to communicate and verify reality, hence communication is distorted and blocked. It also severs us from our divine source of unconditional love and support.

The Adversary makes false promises.

This is part of the second parameter of the state of captivity—acts of perceived kindness. In Chapter 2, I described the many forms that love-bombing and idealization can take and how it causes people to extend their trust to abusers. This often involves flattery, making false promises of security, love, money, fame, success, or whatever other desire can be distorted for control over the target.

When alternated with threats of fear and devaluation, the perceived acts of kindness cause the intermittent reinforcement that keeps people investing more and working harder to maintain the favor of the perpetrators in order to get the occasional rewards and praise. I described the power of false hope to keep people investing their physical, emotional, mental, social, and spiritual capital in relationships and situations, much like people continuing to put money into slot machines, hoping *this will be the time* it finally works out.

Eldredge also states that the Adversary continually terrorizes with fear and false accusations: "Next comes propaganda…the Enemy is constantly broadcasting messages to try to demoralize us…he is constantly putting his spin on things."[27]

This corresponds to the third parameter of the state of captivity—perceived life threats. In Chapter 3, I described what happens when fear is weaponized and how it corrupts the human operating system. Intense fear collapses our energy field and shuts down the autonomic nervous system. This traps people in states of collapse, dissociation and, functional freeze.

Eventually the target ends up believing there's no way out of the situation and pain, so the path of least resistance is to comply and outsource one's power. This is the fourth parameter of the state of captivity—the perceived inability to escape. In Chapter 4, I explained how perpetrators use goal post moving to make their targets believe that the abuse will stop if they just do what they're told. I also emphasized that compliance never ends the abuse. It only prolongs the pain and torture.

Spiritual warfare leaves the target in a state of learned helplessness and spiritual bankruptcy. It's a despair-like state of faithlessness and emptiness. Eventually, as this goes on over time, people become so debilitated and exhausted that they can't even consider the possibility of a way out or a path to freedom.

The surrender into victim consciousness might become so disempowering that it leads people to the point where they can't even meet their basic needs of food, clothing, and shelter. That can cause further feelings of shame, scarcity, self-pity, and downward spirals.

You might have had situations or relationships in your life when you felt like everything was out of your control and you couldn't rescue yourself from your life circumstances. That often causes people to turn to a rescue fantasy, hoping that someone else is going to save them from their feelings of loneliness or their life predicament. It also leads people to hope for someone to save the country or world. Maybe this is how you have felt since 2020.

The first hurdle to exiting the state of captivity is *recognizing that it's not love or care*. The person or people deploying these tactics, whether they're aware of what they're doing or not, are not acting *for your own good*. At this stage, it's about facing the external truth.

This step is part of the awakening. Many people confuse the awareness of abuse with healing. But that's a myth. Awareness is the first step to change, but without taking aligned action, nothing will change, and the person will stay stuck in a state of captivity, even after leaving the abusive relationship or situation.

The second hurdle, which is perhaps even stickier, is the emotional attachment to the injustice. This is when a victim is obsessively thinking about all the injustices done to him. The mind gets stuck in rumination loops, churning on constant thoughts about the injustice, and blaming those who caused the harm. Negative feelings become the lens through which a person sees life. It feels like there's no way to move forward until there's justice for what was done.

It's so easy to get stuck in the victimhood where we try to find power by calling out the abusers and what they did. While that's legitimate on the one hand, on the other hand, it places the locus of control outside ourselves. That's not power. Empowerment comes from *within*, returning the locus of control and agency to ourselves.

Over time, the ongoing state of powerlessness can become woven into a person's identity—how he sees himself and what's possible for him based on that story. Feeling victimized becomes the standard operating system and the person forgets how to access his power. In the case of childhood abuse and neglect, it's possible that many never even knew what it's like to be empowered.

The trap of victimhood

Over time, as the inner state of captivity progresses like an infection, people will likely develop habits of self-sabotage and self-destruction. These get triggered as soon as something reminds their nervous system and subconscious of the unresolved past where it felt like there's no escape. It's usually automatic and happens without our awareness, so it seems like it's out of our control.

In this state, you'll find yourself dimming your light and settling for less than you're worth. Eventually the toxic, negative mindset will turn into resentment and bitterness. That's usually directed toward other people and yourself. You become your own worst enemy. The voice of the perpetrator becomes internalized and you end up treating yourself as you were treated by the one or ones who hurt you. It's not fair what happened, yet you're the only one who can do something about it now.

If you don't do the *inner* work, which starts with self-honesty and owning 100 percent responsibility for yourself and your choices, you'll have a very high probability of repetition. I'm speaking from decades of experience in my own life and through observing so many other cases. I would love others to be able to learn from my mistakes so they can save themselves a lot of time and suffering.

For some, the repetition after abuse may mean going back to past partnerships, friendships, or family members, or continuing to find new abusers in different situations and circumstances while it's the same old story. For others, the victimhood patterns could show up more at work or in other compartmentalized aspects of life.

The longer you stay stuck in the state of captivity and the victimhood consciousness, the more likely the changes in your personality because you start to believe the lies you were taught about yourself. When we make spiritual agreements with these lies, such as *you're unworthy*, that's like a portal that opens to the dark forces. A barrage of more propaganda comes through and before we know it, we become oppressed and feel like we deserve it.

The further down into the pit of false accusations that you allow yourself to go (and sometimes this is through your thoughts), the more you'll turn to unhealthy coping mechanisms and self-destructive behaviors, hoping to fix things. Eventually you'll become a shell of the person you once were. Sometimes others will notice this before you do. This is amplified at the societal level when most of us are living in a state of captivity.

You can tell you're in the victim consciousness by the way you talk to yourself and how you narrate your reality and experiences. For example, if I say *everything happens for a reason*, what do you think?

People coming from the victim perspective could be upset, feel unfairly blamed, or might even get angry and lash out because they don't like the circumstances of their life and they feel like it's their fault or someone else's fault.

People coming from an empowered or thriving state of consciousness might respond with a sense of gratitude even for the challenging times because of how those experiences helped them to shift, grow, and evolve.

One response involves a negative outlook focusing on blame and shame. The other is a positive outlook focusing on gratitude and growth. These are very different responses to the same statement, which implies neither a positive or a negative connotation.

Perspective is reality. Remember, the state of captivity feels real, but the prison bars are holographic. What matters is your perception.

Captivity as a state of consciousness means that you eventually become the prisoner *and* the guard. The abuse conditions you to become your own captor—even long after the perpetrator is gone. This is why abuse is so insidious. It installs a spiritual virus that corrupts your operating system and gets you to abuse and destroy yourself.

The state of captivity is an inner state. It won't just go away when:

- You leave the abuser or situation,
- The truth comes out about the abuser and what happened,
- Justice is served, or
- The abuser is dead.

Physical distance from abusive people and situations helps a lot. It's a great boundary to protect your healing process, whenever possible. But the distance won't get you out of that inner state and it won't stop you from falling into another similar situation. Boundaries are very important, yet they're not the same as healing.

The only way to heal and prevent it from happening again is to *do the inner work.*

Part Two of this book will delve into the liberation of souls to help you start resolving the past so you can move forward. These insights will be applicable to life in the post-2020 world as well as our personal lives. It's all connected. But first I want to plant some seeds for thought and give a bird's eye view of what to look out for so that we don't fall victim to any further captivity campaigns.

Liberating yourself from victimhood starts by facing the truth. The truth is the light that starts to illuminate the darkness.

Initially the acceptance of truth is external—about the perpetrators. That means you figure out what they're doing and start finding the language to explain what they did.

The next part is the more challenging step. It's the internal truth, which means facing your own choices and participation in your life. *This is the only place you'll find your power.* It will lead to deeper self-knowledge and greater self-empowerment.

You're going to need to be willing to see things about yourself that you don't want to see. Self-honesty is the step many people don't reach because they can't bear to face the mistakes they've made or how they're sabotaging what they really want in life. Self-honesty is like confession for Catholics, or the first step in a twelve-step program. First, we have to admit and acknowledge what we are participating in so we can do something to change it.

It's much easier to put all the blame or judgment on someone else. That's why there are cultural and political movements dedicated to celebrating victimhood and promoting it as a lifestyle for the benefit of sympathy and entitlements. This keeps society disempowered and dysfunctional, and that only benefits the perpetrators in the world.

The abuse was never your fault. However, once you wake up and get out, at that point you're the only one keeping yourself in a state of captivity. Technically, it's not *you*—it's your programming. The awesome thing is that you have the power to reprogram yourself.

Staying in the state of captivity will mean sacrificing your dreams in life. You'll talk yourself out of aiming for what you want, such as love, partnership, business, abundance, family, or other success. Or you'll want a dream so badly, but you'll continually run into problems due to the people that you choose to be around and the kinds of situations and habits you get involved with, so it will keep falling apart and adding to the sense of injustice. You'll spend your lifetime blaming others and thinking it's all their fault that you aren't living the life you want, and that will alternate with feelings of self-blame and shame.

That's the path of disempowerment, and it's not fun. Believe me, I was in it for decades and it was a miserable existence. Then I went back into it in the early 2020s when the global events triggered unresolved trauma from my childhood and earlier adult life. I got so focused on what the perpetrators were doing to us that I forgot that's not where my power is.

The greatest gift of the global tyranny was that it forced me to go back into the victim consciousness and understand it at a deeper level. That motivated me to clean up the rubble of the past and turn it into gold, so I could empower and liberate myself, and inspire others to do the same.

What if we don't deal with it?

There's an enormous sacrifice for staying in the state of captivity. The long-term impact is ongoing, even after a person manages to escape the abusive relationship or situation. On a societal level, we haven't escaped the situation per se, even though the pressure to comply with COVID measures has mostly disappeared.

Yet even now, in 2025, we hear public officials and unelected figures at the World Health Organization as well as other global organizations continuing to use aggressive language and threats against "anti-vaxxers" and "conspiracy theorists" who are blamed for stopping people from keeping up with their boosters.

While most people are no longer playing that game, I don't think it's because they woke up and healed the underlying problems that made them susceptible to such manipulation. It's merely because there is currently no social, economic, and psychological pressure to comply. Many people are just one fear campaign and rescue fantasy away from doing it again (whatever the next *it* is) because they're in the state of captivity and don't realize it.

Victimhood is a stage, not a life sentence—it's a state of consciousness, not an identity.

Over the years, I've watched many people become trapped in victimhood. The title of victim becomes part of their identity. It can be enticing to the wounded ego to want sympathy and validation from others about the suffering and injustices endured. We hear plenty of political campaigns promoting victimhood narratives that prey on people's legitimate pain while keeping them trapped there with promises of victim entitlements.

Alternatively, sometimes people get stuck in narratives like "We aren't victims and there's no such thing as trauma." This is a form of denial. None of us gets through life without trauma. When people say they had a great childhood, that's often a sign of emotional neglect. It's a subtle trauma that doesn't look outwardly traumatic and is often minimized as *culture*: "That's just how things were done back then." While that's true, neglect and other traumatic experiences that were minimized leave deep scars on the soul and usually cause a person to adapt through avoidance behaviors, which causes challenges with relationships, money, and life in general.

The victim perspective is black and white, all or nothing. There's no nuance. The expanded truth is nuanced. For example, it's not your fault if you were abused—*and* you're the only one who can do something about it now. Both of these are true. However, a person in a victim state of consciousness will agree with the first one but feel like the second one is a form of blaming the victim. It's not about blaming. It's about self-responsibility and returning the locus of control within, which is the only path out of victimhood. Healing and growing up leads to more nuanced perspectives and truths.

If you recognize that you're currently in a state of captivity to some degree, it doesn't always have to be like this for you. It may feel like there's no escape. That's just how it feels right now. When your perspective shifts, *everything* starts to change.

Beware: There will be a temptation from the ego to hold on to the victimhood because it's easier to stay where you are than to take responsibility for your life and change it. That's why most people stay in the victim consciousness after awakening to the external truth.

You will not experience true freedom and empowerment without owning 100 percent responsibility over your life and your choices.

Authentic freedom isn't just about leaving the abusive person or situation. It's about doing the inner work to clear the old programs and emotional residue, rebuilding self-worth, growing up, and integrating the past in order to open new possibilities and create a new future.

When you take full responsibility for yourself, you'll feel empowered to change your life circumstances and it will be worth it. Your power is in your choices. Yet the challenge is that it doesn't feel like a choice when we are reacting automatically from subconscious programming, which is what happens when we have unresolved trauma.

Tips for opting out of abusive dynamics:

- Do not give into the demands of abusers and tyrants. That will not appease them, no matter how convincing they are when they make promises otherwise. They will keep moving the goal posts, demanding more and more until they drain you dry.
- If you've already complied, but you don't want to anymore, remind yourself that sometimes in life we make mistakes. In those cases, you'll need to be willing to accept that it's time to cut your losses and grieve what was lost. This will involve processing your regrets with compassion, so that you don't continue to beat yourself up for not knowing better and not making better decisions when you didn't have the awareness to do so.
- Make conscious, intentional choices about what you want for yourself and your life in the long-term. That's how you can invest in the present for a better future. Be careful not to sacrifice your long-term peace, health, and other core values for the instant gratification or temporary relief of anxiety, fear, and pain that comes with compliance or escapism.
- Clearly define the terms and conditions of your life. If not, you'll end up complying with, and consenting to, things you regret later. Write down a list of your limits, your non-negotiable boundaries, so that you can use these as filters for what you will and will not accept in relationships and life.
- Set boundaries to protect what matters to you. It's not easy to enforce boundaries with manipulators because they don't take no for an answer. They will try to bulldoze your boundaries or use more sophisticated tactics like guilt-tripping, pity ploys, and snake-tongued sweet-talking. This is why you need to define your non-negotiables *ahead of time*.
- Recognize that your boundaries are first and foremost with yourself. Don't expect other people to respect your boundaries if you don't respect yourself. When you respect yourself and stand by your boundaries, it's easy to walk away when others aren't respecting you or your boundaries.

- Understand that the only way to practice holding firm to your boundaries is in the moment when you're being tested to draw the line. We all learn to manage our boundaries in real time. If you make a mistake and compromise one of your boundaries, you can use that as a learning opportunity.
- Reflect on a moment when you wish you had made a different decision. Envision yourself making that choice instead. This isn't for the purpose of beating yourself up, but for learning from the past. By visualizing your future self making better choices, it's easier to do that next time because this becomes part of your self-concept.
- Keep enforcing your boundaries when tested and you'll notice how your self-worth rises every time. Self-worth is an important immunity from abuse and manipulation.

CHAPTER 6

THE GREATEST DECEPTION

Anti-Life Programming

Covert abuse conditions us to self-sacrifice for the collective. Many of us were taught or programmed by family, religion, and culture that it's noble to sacrifice our values, health, wellbeing, resources, and worthiness *for the greater good.*

This is parasitic manipulation programming that conditions people to sacrifice themselves for others, as if it's the empathic and compassionate thing to do.

That program leads to being controlled by external forces and allowing others to take advantage of us. It traps people in the ancestral legacy of trauma, feeling guilty for wanting to set healthy boundaries or for healing and thriving in life. Essentially, the goal is to make you forget how powerful you are.

Dr. Gabor Maté wrote a book called *When the Body Says No* and he speaks of this topic in videos and interviews. Maté highlights the obituaries of people who died of cancer, heart disease, and other ailments, drawing attention to how they were described as *having lived their life selflessly for others.*

Those obituaries reflect the cultural values that praise people for their self-sacrifice, an act that contributes to chronic illness and early death. They sacrificed their own health and life by putting others first. This is not a virtue. It's an anti-life program that feeds parasites. It leads to morbidity and death.

If you want to heal and thrive, you'll need to unsubscribe from this programming. As Maté emphasizes, *if you don't say no, your body will say no for you.*

A life of self-sacrifice leads to the corruption of values, victimhood, rage, resentment, regret, unhappiness, toxicity, codependence, depression, chronic illness, and early death.

Do you believe you're allowed to be healthier and happier than your family (or other people around you)? Really pause and reflect on that for a moment. Many people feel like they have to sacrifice their happiness and health when those around them are suffering. This can lead people to believe that it's selfish to set boundaries and feel like they don't have the right to be well when others aren't. Sacrificing your health doesn't make sick people healthier, it just makes you sick, too.

Your boundaries are first and foremost with yourself. These define the limits of what you will and won't do, what you will and won't accept, what is and what is not okay for you. Your boundaries protect your values, health, self-worth, wealth, and wellbeing. You're allowed to prioritize your health and wellbeing, even if others around you aren't healthy or well.

Your boundaries are your responsibility to manage. This may seem unfair at first if you're still struggling to release the distorted programming that you received in childhood. You might have the fantasy that people should know how to behave and respect others. In an ideal world that would be true, but this is not reality. Knowing how and when to say no is a crucial boundary.

Are you starting to notice some of the ways that your family, workplace, culture, and society promote self-sacrifice?

It makes for a potent propaganda campaign. If you feel ashamed for unknowingly subscribing to your family's gaslighting around the self-sacrifice programming, remember that in recent years, nearly 80 percent of society fell for the biggest gaslighting campaign in the history of humanity. This shows us how disempowered the human race is and how easy it is for us to be manipulated. We can acknowledge this with compassion and without blame, shame, and judgment.

It's incredibly common to be manipulated by an anti-life deception campaign while thinking that you're doing the right thing. If you fall or fell into this trap in any area of your life, it could be helpful to reflect on who taught you to abandon yourself to make others feel good. When did that start? And how did it serve you?

It probably had something to do with feeling safe. If you don't identify the origin and benefit of that distortion program, it will continue running in the background and you could fall for it again.

Don't beat yourself up about having subscribed to this program. It wasn't your fault. The important thing is that your eyes are opening now, and you can make new choices and transform your life moving forward. This is your responsibility.

Notice what happens when someone tries to force or coerce you into doing something that's not okay with you. What if he implies that you're selfish or not a good person if you don't do what he wants? That's where it gets tricky.

If you're in a low-frequency state of guilt, despair, hopelessness, helplessness, fear, and shame, you're a prime target for predators and parasites to use this against you.

If you're in a high-frequency state of consciousness, you won't be so easily swayed to comply or prove your worth to others because you'll *know* that you're worthy. You'll have access to your critical thinking, intuition, insights, creativity, and imagination, as well as the courage to set boundaries and protect what matters to you.

Your consciousness determines your perspective, the inner resources available to you, and the choices you make. Your state of consciousness creates your reality.

When public health is used to defile personal liberty

If we analyze how this same pattern was underlying the Nazi campaign in Germany nearly one hundred years ago, we can see eerily similar messaging in the campaign for public health and sacrificing for the greater good.

When people dismiss the current parallels to Nazi Germany, it's because they lack perspective. They're comparing the final product (concentration camps, torture, mass murder) with what we are seeing in the world right now.

Abuse doesn't start how it ends. It gets there in gradual steps.

It makes sense that many people have this limited perspective because that's the only part I remember hearing about in history class, too. They didn't teach us about the escalation over time of gradually increasing public health policies, narrative spinning, and violations against human rights that laid the groundwork for such a thing to happen years after it started.

The dehumanization and demonization of minorities began via public health campaigns.

The Nazis were able to convince doctors to accept that Jews were a source of "biologic degeneration." Their "racial hygiene" agenda included—together with the Jews—the disabled, the mentally ill, those with diseases like tuberculosis and STDs, as well as gypsies, dissidents, artists, intellectuals, thought leaders, and people of different ethnic backgrounds.

The Nazis started promoting the ideology that these people were diseased and dangerous. They had already been indoctrinating doctors and medically trained academics into their eugenics science for decades before that.

Eugenicists aim to control the human population by promoting reproduction among those with certain characteristics while sterilizing or euthanizing the "undesirables" under the guise of improving the human race.

The fact that that the Nazis got doctors to go along with this public health campaign ought to reveal how easy it is to manipulate medical experts and those who are entrusted with the wellbeing of people—those who took an oath *to do no harm*—to do harm disguised as good.

Volksgesundheit (public health—literally: health of the people) was positioned as priority over individual autonomy, life, and liberty in health care. This ideology justified unlimited medical atrocities and abuse of human rights.

By the late 1930s, Nazis were banning Jews from public places, even in Nazi-occupied areas abroad, like restaurants, cafés, bars, theaters, cinemas, concert halls, museums, libraries, swimming pools and other sports venues, and parks. They started persecuting Jews as well as dissidents, artists, and thought leaders who opposed what was happening.

Does this sound familiar?

Of course, during COVID, the campaign was much more covert and sophisticated. The government and media weren't openly talking about eugenics and *racial hygiene*. That's already been played and would be too obvious. But we can recognize the same intention in the subtext of the public health campaign.

Dehumanization, segregation, and apartheid are dangerous. These ideologies, and the public policies that enforce them, inevitably lead to the same atrocities. They are always couched in "public health" or other seemingly noble "scientific" justifications. The more covert tactics of using collectivist phrases, such as *for the greater good*, simply makes the tyranny easier for people to swallow.

Sometime in early 2022, just like that, it all got swept under the rug as if it had never happened. *But it did happen*.

Right now, it might seem like everything is fine because the COVID campaign appeared to disappear. Yet it is mind-blowing that we aren't talking about what happened and how it's still affecting us while the narrative is pivoting to the next thing, and the next.

We are still hearing open calls for more information control and censorship. The control campaign is not over. The pieces are being moved in the background while most people aren't paying attention because they'd like to forget the nightmare of the early 2020s. That's understandable—however, the perpetrators are still pushing forward their agendas.

There are always red flags of abuse before it gets bad. The tricky part is to recognize the warning signs before it gets to that point. That's even more challenging during the moments of seeming calm and the temporary respite from the intensity of the abuse cycle.

People often judge abuse survivors for not leaving sooner. I think that many people around the world are currently in the process of learning the hard way why abuse victims don't leave before it gets bad. *It doesn't look like abuse at first.*

It may sometimes seem obvious to an outsider that another person is being abused. But it's not so obvious to the person who is in it.

Likewise, the same can happen to a society. It's easy to look back at history from the outside and feel morally superior to those who enabled such a thing as the Nazi regime, but we have the advantage of retrospect. I think the answer is becoming clear now how such a thing could have happened in Germany.

One day, future generations will judge us for the roles we are playing right now. What will you tell them when they ask what you did during times of tyranny?

Many times in human history, people have been faced with growing tyranny and they had to choose whether to stand up for their individual liberties and human rights, or to comply with the abuse in order to gain a sense of safety. Both paths are risky.

Which future do you prefer for you, your children, and grandchildren?

Your body is your autonomous zone

You have the right to decide what you put in your body and not, what you consent to and not. You have the right to refuse medical treatment, even if it's life-saving.

This was the most important standard of human rights that came from the Nuremberg Code. It was written after World War II because the Nazis had conducted heinous medical experiments on human beings. They experimented, tortured, imprisoned, and murdered specific groups of humans, all in the name of "science."

Now, looking back, we can see that it wasn't science. It was ideology—collective delusional psychosis and cult fanaticism that people were conditioned to accept as normal and for the good of the nation. As we explored earlier in this chapter, the Nazis even brainwashed the doctors to comply with their ideology of racial hygiene.

This is why those who wrote the Nuremberg Code determined that: "The voluntary consent of the human subject is absolutely essential." It's interesting how they didn't write human *being*—they wrote human *subject*, as if to emphasize that medical experiments had been conducted. It was a subtle yet important clue for societies in the future.

Of course, we ought to acknowledge that the version of the Nuremberg Code we read today was likely meticulously curated by the propagandists of that time. Still, it tells us, without directly telling us, what happened.

To dismiss the Nuremberg Code is to stand against human rights. Remember this when you hear people smearing the Nuremberg Code and trying to say it doesn't apply now because *this* time, it's *really* about public health. That's an incredibly naive lens through which to view history, and the repetitive playbook of tyrants disguising themselves as the heroes of public health and the human race.

Consent is our choice as individuals.

The law of consent is related to self-determination, the freedom to control your body, mind, and spirit. It is not a result of legislation but of inherent rights that a human being has by birthright. It is also known as natural or cosmic law.

Remember the power of your choice and the right to bodily autonomy when you hear the social and political pressure (bribing, shaming, blaming, and guilt-tripping) to do something to your body that you are not okay with. Keep in mind, the perpetrators will always try to make you feel like a bad person if you don't do it.

They'll aim to make you feel like you don't have the right or the worth to make your own choice because your individuality is not valid when it comes to *the greater good*. You're expected to sacrifice your own wellbeing or life for the collective.

Millions of people in history have been killed as a result of ideologies using the euphemism *for the greater good.* They probably thought their situation was the exception, too, just like every abuse victim wants to believe that her partner is the exception to the red flags of abuse.

The moral code of cannibalism

Abusers expect their targets to sacrifice themselves to meet the abuser's needs and whims. They have very creative and covert ways of tricking people into this because they need our consent, lest they resort to revealing their true nature through desperate force.

In covert abusive families and social systems, if you don't consent to sacrificing yourself, they sacrifice you. The abusers program you to destroy yourself before others destroy you. In a distorted way, the act of self-sacrifice is a way of feeling some control over a powerless, hopeless situation. This is why it's so easy to give into the anti-life cult programming. Self-sabotage happens gradually but quickly.

Ayn Rand described self-sacrifice as the morality of an *anti-life philosophy*.

In the early twentieth century, terms like "covert narcissist" didn't exist. Yet Ayn Rand described in her novel *Atlas Shrugged*, with an incredible richness and precision of language, these personalities and their motives. She described them from the bottom to the top of the hierarchy in society, revealing the tactics of *those who expect others to voluntarily consent to victimization for the greater good.*

Rand wrote about a fictional society of people who didn't want to take responsibility for their lives. People wanted other people to decide and do for them so that they could remain blameless and only invest the most minimal effort in life while waiting for someone else to solve their problems.

Corrupt, mediocre, and entitled "looters" were in power. Society was collapsing. It was a time of *an endless, temporary, national emergency.* Sounds familiar, doesn't it?

The few people who were willing to take responsibility were endlessly persecuted as sinners by the "moochers," those who condemned others for making money, while feeling entitled to live off their efforts and resources. Talk about cognitive dissonance!

At another level, the corrupt "looters" in government were pocketing as much as they could, while creating more and more unjust laws and absurd federal regulations, further exacerbating the destruction and collapse of society—all the while saying it was *for the greater good.*

They used euphemistic language such as "equality" to restrain the efforts of those in society who still had the willingness to accept responsibility and the drive to build and contribute value to the infrastructure of the country.

The responsible and capable people were publicly shamed because others felt inferior instead of being grateful for trains, bridges, buildings, electricity, and other things that made the country functional. The cardinal sin of an individual in Rand's fictional society was to create or produce anything of value without sacrificing it all for others.

The looters and moochers constantly congratulated themselves on their moral superiority as they put on exaggerated and hypocritical displays of virtue signaling. Their dystopian social system demanded that people consent to self-sacrifice through the weaponization of false guilt and fear.

Rand described "the sanction of the victim," whereby a person voluntarily consents (albeit as a result of distress due to the coercion, persecution, and deceit of others) to being victimized by *sacrificing oneself for the greed or need of another.*

This went on for some time as the infrastructure continued to collapse until a few brave people stood up upon being targeted and persecuted. They decided *to accept no unearned guilt* and chose to peacefully strike against the societal demands for martyrdom, which Rand called the code of "moral cannibalism."

One of the main characters in *Atlas Shrugged* is Henry Rearden, an entrepreneur married to a woman who's completely subscribed to the code of moral cannibalism. She was constantly putting her husband down, minimizing his hard work, shaming him for his success and tireless efforts to keep making his important contribution to society.

Of course, she also found great pleasure in his money and the status it awarded her in society.

Rearden produced a proprietary metal that was needed to build strong bridges and railroads, forming an important backbone of the infrastructure in the country. His efforts were continually thwarted by his family, which was rooting for his demise, as well as by the government.

Throughout the book, Rearden starts to understand what's happening in society and why it's collapsing. Gaining macro-to-micro vision, he also begins to see the covert evil in his wife, mother, and brother more clearly. Against their wishes, he refuses to consent to being victimized by the system when he is called to trial for not giving away his business and the intellectual copyright to his metal.

They realized he was going to vanish like the other great men and women who had gone on strike. This meant that all his assets would be confiscated by the corrupt government as a punishment for this act of dissidence, leaving his family penniless. That's when Rearden finally saw their true colors, in what Rand described as "the concerto of deliverance."

In a spectacular revelation, after standing up for his values and refusing to consent to victimizing himself through the act of self-immolation during the trial, Rearden finally understands his wife's motivation all along:

> The lust that drives others to enslave an empire, had become, in her limits, a passion for power over him. She had set out to break him, as if, unable to equal his value, she could surpass it by destroying it, as if the measure of his greatness would thus become the measure of hers, as if—he thought with a shudder—as if the vandal who smashed a statue were greater than the artist who had made it.
>
> He remembered her hammering derision of his work.... Her line of attack, which he had found so baffling, had been constant and clear—it was his self-esteem she had sought to destroy, knowing that a man who surrenders

> his value is at the mercy of anyone's will; it was his moral purity she had struggled to breach, it was his confident rectitude she had wanted to shatter by means of the poison of guilt—as if, were he to collapse, his depravity would give her a right to hers.
>
> For the same purpose and motive, for the same satisfaction, as others weave complex systems of philosophy to destroy generations, or establish dictatorships to destroy a country, so she, possessing no weapons except femininity, had made it her goal to destroy one man.[28]

Again, Rand's description is *eerily* similar to the political and cultural movements we've witnessed in society in recent years. Many of those who recognized these dangerous trends in our culture had already experienced the same in relationships and family.

It's crucial to understand that this act of self-immolation requires our consent. Rearden's wife sought to destroy his self-esteem in order to gain control over him, which is one of the most important clues nowadays as we face an unprecedented assault on our human rights in the name of *the greater good.*

Our self-worth is not meant to depend on other people, on what they think of us or how they treat us. Self-worth means it comes from *within* the self. That's why abusers always aim to destroy the target's self-worth. I'll go more in depth on self-worth as our greatest immunity to abuse and tyranny in Chapter 14.

The pressure to fit in

It can be tricky when you know something to be true while others are telling you that you're crazy or wrong. They might directly say or imply that everyone else is fine with it or everybody sees it differently, so *you're the only one with the problem.*

That could cause you to doubt yourself because it's you vs. groupthink. You could assume that the group must know better than you, because, rationally speaking, it's more unlikely that you're the one who's right and all of them are wrong. Yet that's often not the case in a social system involving an abusive person (or an abusive hierarchy of people) and their enablers.

Many of the enablers are good people, however they lack the awareness, willingness, or courage to see the truth, so they defend the system. Usually that's because they have a dependence on the abuser or the abusive system. It could be a financial, emotional, logistical, or other form of dependence, such as status or the illusion they want to believe in, such as the perfect family. They're getting a need met, so they'll defend the abuser and fight to maintain the abusive system—no matter how unhealthy or dysfunctional it is.

The system is designed to defend the system.

As humans we have a biological need to feel accepted and connected to others. That's why abuse dynamics have even more sway in a group context.

In the 1950s, Solomon Asch did social experiments to demonstrate the power of group conformity. He placed several actors in a group with one participant who didn't know that the others were told to give the wrong answer to the question on purpose.

Upon viewing pictures of lines, the participants were asked which line was longer. The actors were told to give their incorrect answers first. Asch found that 35 percent of the participants followed the opinion of the actors, even when the answer was wrong.

The Asch conformity experiments were done with American male students. More recently, it was questioned whether the same results would be found in other demographics and locations. So, the Asch study was replicated in other countries—with similar results.

One of the replication studies was done in 2023 with more than 200 participants, concluding: "Our study provides further evidence that the influence of groups on individuals' judgments is a universal phenomenon, and is still valid today."[29]

The 2023 study expanded to also include political opinions and discovered the following:

> Moreover, our study suggests that group pressure is not only influential in the simple line task but also when it comes to political opinions. We randomized the groups' response to five different political statements and find an average conformity rate of 38%. Hence, these results suggest that the original finding of Asch can also be generalized to matters of opinion.[30]

The study authors noted that all subjects in the experiment were strangers, and the authors questioned if the results would differ if the group pressure involved friends or family. That's indeed a good question.

This phenomenon played out in families and groups of friends during the COVID campaign's absurd, irrational, and harmful mandates. Social media was absolutely necessary for that campaign to work. The global mafia needed people to do their bidding by applying social pressure within their network of extended family and friends.

The need for social approval is rooted in a need for safety. We are wired this way. This goes back to our earliest tribal origins. Humans are pack creatures. Conformity is a survival mechanism.

While we are also individuals, and our individuality is important; we don't exist in a vacuum. We exist in social systems. For this reason, to understand the individual, we must also take consider the environment in which that person lives. This can include aspects of the physical surroundings, such as country and local culture. It also includes the mental, emotional, social, technological, and spiritual environment of the person.

The social environment is the social system—the partner, family, workplace, friends, community, and society at large. Nowadays, it also includes online groups and "communities." These are layers of social systems, expanding from the micro level to the macro level.

A social system is made up of individuals who maintain the status quo of that system. It takes on system dynamics, where no matter how dysfunctional it is, people will often defend it and attack those who threaten the status quo.

One of the biggest threats to any abusive social system is the person who speaks up about abuse. When you disclose the abuse in a family, workplace, or other social system, the others often instantly turn on you. They'll launch *ad hominem* attacks against you, otherwise known as smear campaigns, in order to defend the system.

You'll hear all kinds of rationalizations, justifications, and minimizations to get you to stop speaking the truth and instead give the abuser the benefit of the doubt:

"That didn't happen."

"Nobody is perfect."

"You aren't perfect, either."

"It was a joke."

"They really care about you in their own way."

"Just give them a chance."

"This time it will be different."

That's why we heard similar propaganda in the COVID narrative:

"It's about science."

"Wearing a mask is like wearing pants."

"I'm not wearing my mask for me, I'm wearing it for you."

"We are all in this together."

"Staying apart keeps us together."

It was highly incentivized to do what the majority is doing, lest you meet the wrath of those who wanted you to conform to make themselves feel safer. We heard plenty of *ad hominem* attacks to silence and discredit people:

"You're anti-vax."

"You're anti-science."

"You're a conspiracy theorist."

"You're spreading fear."

"You're dangerous and out of line."

"Stay in your lane, you're not an expert."

Agenda 2030: The Greatest Deception

The World Economic Forum (WEF) tells us that by 2030, "You'll own nothing and you'll be happy." That sure sounds like flatlined equality among us peasants, while the global mafia gather all the monopoly money and property for themselves until they own everything.

Of course, they sprinkle it with feel-good words like "equality" and "sustainability," along with assurances that they'll rent us what we need. But these are also the people calling for information control, a net zero carbon footprint (remember, humans exhale carbon dioxide), and the implementation of globally recognized digital medical records for vaccinations and travel.

These are not conspiracy theories, as some might think. Well-known public officials are openly discussing all these topics during the WEF meetings, and those videos are available online.

They always tell us what they're doing. But are we listening?

If we add one and one, it's clear that they only want to give us access to goods and services that we earn through behavioral compliance with the social credit system connected to a digital ID.

Do you remember consenting to The Great Reset? Neither do I. But this dystopian future will be ours if we don't withdraw our consent sooner rather than later.

They will justify continually increasing levels of abuse of human rights and individual sovereignty, while claiming to be upholding democracy and human rights. This is their covert campaign template, which they will copy and paste from crisis to crisis (read: opportunity) for their increased dominance of the world.

We're already several years into the *decade of transformation.* Most people are sleepwalking into it as the technocracy is gradually being imposed upon us as a pre-determined solution to the global and local crises.

Yet it requires our consent. This is our human right and responsibility. We have innate worth as well as the right to choose bodily autonomy and individual sovereignty. This is the part they don't want us to realize because this is where we find our power.

They intend for us to feel like there's no escape, that there's no option but compliance and dependence. They will continue telling us that self-sacrifice is a necessary evil for the greater good. Remember, this is an anti-life program based on the morality of cannibalism.

The individual *and* the collective are important.

It's not a question of "or." The collective is formed by the individuals. When individuals are well, the collective is well. Therefore, individual wellbeing is the foundation of societal wellbeing.

Societal health and wellbeing starts with the individual. If society is sick, it's because individuals are not well. If society is at war, it's because individuals are at war with themselves. If lies rule a society, it's because we as individuals are lying to ourselves.

The remedy is not found in collectivist ideologies and spiritual bypassing, but in the hearts and minds of individuals who willingly take responsibility for their own lives. This involves paying attention to what we are consenting to, withdrawing our consent where we need to, speaking the truth with those who want to listen, then working on healing ourselves from the harm and injustices done so we can create the life we want to live, and the world we want to pass on to future generations.

Through the inner work, individuals start to thrive and naturally feel driven to *voluntarily* contribute something of value to the collective. *That* leads to a thriving society.

When people aren't well and instead are stuck in survival states, they don't have the energy or ability to contribute to something beyond themselves. In that state, the focus is self-preservation. It's very common after trauma to unknowingly become self-centered and entitled in order to survive because we can get stuck in primal states of defensiveness and dependence.

When individuals are disempowered and desperate for self-preservation, they often become parasitic and take from others—by force or coercion—what's not theirs. This creates violations and win-lose situations. *This is how victims can become perpetrators.*

The contribution that an integrated, thriving individual offers the collective is something given voluntarily, not through a violation of consent. This voluntary contribution, in turn, provides a sense of value exchange and fulfillment to the individual and the collective. That creates a win-win situation.

As more of us individuals do the inner work to become healthy and whole, our collective society will also reflect healing and wholeness.

In order to be healthy and whole, it's our responsibility to clearly define our personal core values so that we are not susceptible to a corrupt code of moral cannibalism through outside coercion, threats, or force.

If we are not clear about what matters to us as individuals—and what we ought to protect with our boundaries—all of that will be coerced and taken from us through our own unknowing participation in the social engineering process.

If we consent, under social pressure, to allow our conscience to be violated, our will to be forced, and our God-given individual sovereignty and worth to be stripped away from us, that is how the individual and collective human soul become cannibalized.

The power of choice, to consent or not, is our most basic human right. Choice is where you'll find your power, and that's why abusers want to take away our power to choose.

Remind yourself of your inherent human value. The longer the grooming and abuse goes on, the easier it is to forget that we are sovereign, worthy beings. You have the right to claim autonomy over your body, mind, and soul. Each of us has authority and self-ownership over our own life. This is our divine birthright.

CHAPTER 7

WHAT HAPPENED?

The Violation of Consent

What we witnessed in the early 2020s was an atrocious violation of consent and coerced compliance. It's very similar to what happens in covert abusive relationships and smaller social systems. In this chapter, we will explore these topics more in depth that so we can learn from what happened and prevent it from happening again.

There are both overt and covert forms of violating consent and coercing compliance. Overt perpetrators openly violate a target's right to consent with force like a bulldozer. It's usually pretty easy to recognize them as the bad guys in the movies. The covert ones want to coerce your voluntary consent so they can say it was your choice. They go about this more subtly by telling you it's for your own good and the good of others, therefore implying that if you don't do it, you're a bad person.

Covert perpetrators are the most dangerous because they're so hidden and insidious. The covert form of abuse is the more sophisticated model. It's evil disguised as good. Perhaps this is why Dante Alighieri's *Inferno* put the treacherous, traitors, frauds, and betrayers at the bottom of the pit of Hell—even worse than the violent.

Covert psychopaths are *beings without conscience inhabited by evil entities playing good.* With narcissists, the person's soul is still in negotiation with the evil entity. Sometimes you can see the love of their soul in their eyes, while other times they're gone and it's something else there instead. With psychopaths, their soul is completely gone, and their body is but an empty vehicle for evil entities that camouflage their nature by playing good. Sometimes you'll notice their eyes suddenly appear to turn solid black.

Perhaps this is why psychopathy is a field of study but not a diagnosis. The more overt form—what laymen call sociopathy—is diagnosed as anti-social personality disorder. Maybe the reason why the covert form of psychopathy isn't in the *Diagnostic and Statistical Manual of Psychiatry* is because the fields of medicine and psychology lack the ability to define evil, which is the realm of the spirit.

The covert form is far more dangerous because of how well-disguised it is and how far it can go due to its treacherous nature. By the time the target realizes what's happening, it's usually too late and the damage is done. It's also more challenging for the target to point out what's going on to others. That makes it even more isolating.

Most people don't believe the target because covert abuse is disguised as good. With the exception of some overt forms of violation and force, the COVID campaign was covert abuse and that's why the perpetrators were able to get away with it.

Most therapists aren't able to recognize the covert form of abuse. I've had several therapists from various countries as clients, and they all told me that this type of abuse wasn't part of their training. Hence, these therapists were in covert abusive relationships for decades, unable to see what was happening. Many of my clients had been to therapists to get help for this kind of abuse, only to be gaslit and re-traumatized by the therapists who didn't see what was happening.

Coercive control is one of the main elements of covert abuse. Coercion was used to violate consent and gain compliance on a mass scale during the COVID campaign.

The violation of consent

If we reflect on all that's taken place during the early 2020s and look at the trajectory of where it appears to be going from here, it becomes clear that it was not about a pandemic or public health. It was about the degradation of our most basic human rights disguised as *for the greater good.*

If we get to the very heart of the matter, what we find is the theme of consent. Consent is the power of choice—your natural right to participate in your life, to choose to say yes or no. This is your most basic human right.

The violation of consent isn't always so obvious. What starts off as subtle coercive control can eventually become overt force. The violations of consent usually become more severe as time goes on, unless we stop participating.

If we want to prevent the same covert and overt tyrannical tactics being used for ongoing control agendas, the conversation we ought to have is about restoring and respecting the value of our natural human right to consent.

This could be the topic that unites humans of all different political and ideological stances. It's important that we don't lose sight of this basic human right as the narratives pivot from one crisis to another.

It's essential in relationships and life to remember that *"no" is a complete sentence.*

Sometimes we may feel pressured or expected to give explanations for our boundaries, to defend our right to say no. But when dealing with manipulative characters and their enablers, it's best not to give explanations because those will only be interpreted as openings to negotiate the boundary.

Anytime people push back on your "no," that should be a red flag. Keep in mind that there are both overt and covert forms of pushing back. The overt way is forceful. The covert way is based on emotional manipulation and coercion like trying to make you feel sorry for the perpetrators, to feel guilty about something you're not responsible for, or to shame you as a bad person if you don't do what they want.

Manipulators don't like to hear the word no because it means they're not getting what they want.

In 2021, I made a parody video to highlight the red flags in the COVID vax campaign,[31] inspired by a British campaign called "Tea Consent," which was used as a metaphor to help people to understand sexual consent as if making someone a cup of tea.[32] The same applies to jabs, medical devices, and any other substances and procedures.

Western society has made some growth around the concept of sexual consent in recent decades. Yet it's important to understand that one's right to consent is not merely limited to a sexual context.

Coercive control is abuse

In light of ongoing news trends using language and psychological priming that appears to signal more tyrannical agendas underway, it's important to review the concept of coercive control.

While most people can recognize overt force as abusive, many are not aware of coercive control, which is the more covert form of the violation of boundaries and consent.

Covert psychopaths are adept at tricking people into doing what they want through the meticulous use of coercion tactics. The most sophisticated ones can even get the targets to think it was their own idea!

From interpersonal relationships to family systems, workplaces, social groups, and society at large, the signs of coercive control are very similar. Being able to energetically discern when this is happening is one of the most important life skills you can have so you don't fall into the anti-life programming.

Many people consented under duress to participate in a massive medical experiment during COVID due to the covert violation of consent. That's not true consent. Many people felt it would cause more pain to resist, just like the woman whose husband rapes her. In some cases, people were desperate for something that was being overtly threatened or withheld from them, such as medical treatment or the ability to earn a living, travel, participate in public life, and see loved ones.

Some people believed the experimental injectable was going to save their life because it was promoted as *safe and effective*. Then many people had horrible and debilitating adverse effects or even lost their lives. The injured survivors and bereaved families who lost loved ones have been mostly ignored, dismissed, shamed, and gaslit about it by the authorities and most of society, which is heaping abuse upon abuse.

The same happens in families and other social systems when a victim speaks out about abuse that took place. The enablers don't want to believe it, so they further abuse the victim in order to maintain their perception of reality.

Many people were manipulated into thinking that consenting to the experimental drug technology was the responsible thing to do for others, and if they didn't do their part, because *we're all in it together*, then it's their fault that society can't go back to normal.

Signs of coercive control

- Isolation from friends and family
- Subtle threats or intimidation
- Sabotaging your self-care
- Restricting your mobility
- Financial control
- False guilt
- Shaming

The manipulators' favorite tools to carry out these acts are gaslighting, guilt-tripping, pity ploys, blame-shifting, fear campaigns, goal-post moving, triangulation, future faking, stonewalling, the silent treatment, smear campaigns, minimization, and rationalization.

Coercion is not consent

The first tenet of the Nuremberg Code gives the best definition of coercive control vs. voluntary consent. It can be applied to medical experiments (as indicated by the use of the phrase human *subject*) and just about anything else that a person is asked, expected, required, mandated, compelled, threatened, or intimidated to do. The first tenet reads:

> The voluntary consent of the human subject is absolutely essential. This means that the person involved should have legal capacity to give consent; should be so situated as *to be able to exercise free power of choice, without the intervention of any element of force, fraud, deceit, duress, over-reaching, or other ulterior form of constraint or coercion*; and should have sufficient knowledge and comprehension of the elements of the subject matter involved as to enable him to make an understanding and enlightened decision.[33] (Emphasis added.)

There are some *very* important keywords and phrases used here to help us understand coercive control. You might recognize the above terms as a checklist for all the violations of consent that were used to push the COVID vax on entire populations. You might also recognize how these were used in your personal or professional relationships.

To clarify, *it's for your good* is not an exemption clause for the Nuremberg Code or voluntary consent. That's indeed the exact phrase that nearly every abuser and tyrant ever used to justify his actions or policies.

The reason these terms (in italics) had to be explicitly stated in the Nuremberg Code is because of how easily things can be distorted to violate consent in public health campaigns. We would be wise to recognize that the same concepts can apply to any interpersonal relationship or public campaign.

A law against coercive control

Coercive and controlling behavior is a crime in the UK—but only at home. In 2015, the UK passed a law to protect domestic abuse victims from coercive and controlling behavior.

Yet just a handful of years later, the British government went full on into the coercive control plan with COVID restrictions and vax mandates. Apparently, it's only coercive control in the UK if it's a micro domestic issue at home—because macro domestic issues in society are clearly exempt. That's an interesting application of cognitive dissonance.

The official government website for this law states that victims who experience "extreme psychological and emotional abuse, can bring their perpetrators to justice."[34]

What about all the emotional abuse by politicians, governments, corporations, media, and other institutions to control people by terrifying, coercing, or threatening them into taking the jab and following other mandates that violated their human rights?

The government claims to be sending a message that it's wrong to violate the trust of those closest to you. Does that mean it believes that it's only wrong to violate the trust of people *close* to you and that it's okay to violate the trust of those who aren't close to you? Is that how it justifies the societal level of abuse?

The government website defines coercive control as "a purposeful pattern of incidents that occur over time in order for one individual to exert power, control or coercion over another."[35] That's *exactly* what happened during COVID on a mass scale.

When exposed, the abusers double down

Once the abusers' coercive control is exposed, they predictably have the same response. They'll wash themselves of all accountability for their acts of manipulation and coercion, while flipping it around to blame the victim.

When the target suffers a devastating loss or otherwise gets hurt by complying with the coercive control, the covert abuser will say, "But it was your choice." That's only a partial truth, and it's deception. People got tricked and pressured into consenting. This is a very sick game, and it only works with our participation.

It's no surprise that we are already hearing this phrase deployed by many covert abusers on the global stage as millions of people have been harmed or killed by the mandates and injections or lost their jobs, education, medical care, or the ability to see loved ones and travel if they didn't submit to the jabs.

Each of us is ultimately responsible for the choices we make—and we ought to make those decisions wisely by vetting people and doing independent research. Yet in the case of coercion, a person makes a false choice under duress or deceit. Therefore, it's a violation of basic human rights. It's up to us to set our boundaries and know our rights. Yet we can only do that when we know our worthiness.

For example, during the vax mandates, people were given a false choice or double bind: Get jabbed or else you'll lose your job, education, ability to travel, go to the doctor or hospital, visit loved ones, or even to go to restaurants, bars, concerts, conventions, sports, and other events. Many people didn't want either option, but they were coerced into thinking that those were the *only* options. That's the predicament of every abuse victim who is presented with a double bind.

I'm hearing of more people every week who say their biggest life regret is making the decision to get jabbed, and that they felt deceived into it. And they were. They were pressured and tricked.

Comedian and podcaster Jimmy Dore did a fantastic segment on the criminal liars who said nobody was forced to get a vaccine: "The first lie was the vaccine would stop the transmission and the pandemic. The second lie was we never said the vaccine would stop the transmission and stop the pandemic. Now the third lie is that everyone had a choice and we never made anybody take it."[36]

In that segment with Dore, evolutionary theorist Bret Weinstein adds:

> I think I know how it is that they're telling this lie. What they mean is no one was *physically* forced. They were obviously coerced, threatened, unemployed, if they didn't follow through.
>
> This was all sorted out at Nuremberg. Informed consent was codified at the Nuremberg Court because the Nazi doctors violated a principle that even though it had not been spelled out, the court believed every doctor should understand, which is that not only does the patient have

> a right to refuse any experimental treatment, they have a right to full information about what that treatment is.
>
> The fact is that we were not well-informed, we were lied to. Consent was coerced. That's a double violation of the Nuremberg Code. This is something over which several doctors were literally hanged until dead. That's how important this principle is and we are pretending it never happened. This was an obvious violation, and we ought to remember that.[37]

Tony Blair, the UK's former prime minister, has continued to push the jabs as well as the digitalization of the data on who is vaxxed and who isn't. He also openly promises "a whole slew of new vaccines, injectables, that are going to deal with some of the worst diseases of the world that are going to give us the opportunity to make big changes in the health of the world."[38]

But wait, there's more.

The *philanthropaths* are gearing up for an even stealthier method of violating consent. This time they won't be able to say it was a choice. When they get called out, they will circle back to the *it's for your own good* part.

In a 2022 study, published in *The Oxford Handbook of Intergenerational Ethics* titled "Moral Bioenhancement and Future Generations: Selecting Martyrdom?" the abstract states:

> Moral bioenhancement is a biological modification or intervention which makes moral behavior more likely. There are a number of ways this could potentially be achieved, including pharmaceuticals, non-invasive brain stimulation, or genetic engineering. Moral bioenhancement can be distinguished from other kinds of enhancement because it primarily benefits others, rather than just the individual who has been enhanced. With the challenges that will face future generations, such as climate change and the rise of artificial intelligence, it

> is even more important to address the possibilities of moral bioenhancement.[39]

In a 2019 bioethics study called "Compulsory moral bioenhancement should be covert," the abstract reads:

> Some theorists argue that moral bioenhancement ought to be compulsory. I take this argument one step further, arguing that if moral bioenhancement ought to be compulsory, then its administration ought to be covert rather than overt. This is to say that *it is morally preferable for compulsory moral bioenhancement to be administered without the recipients knowing* that they are receiving the enhancement. My argument for this is that if moral bioenhancement ought to be compulsory, then *its administration is a matter of public health*, and for this reason should be governed by public health ethics. I argue that the covert administration of a compulsory moral bioenhancement program better conforms to public health ethics than does an overt compulsory program. In particular, a covert compulsory program promotes values such as liberty, utility, equality, and autonomy better than an overt program does. Thus, *a covert compulsory moral bioenhancement program is morally preferable to an overt moral bioenhancement program.*[40] (Emphases added.)

That's chilling. This bioethics study openly argues in favor of using public health to *morally* justify the covert administration of biomedical technology to improve a person's moral behavior.

The public health *ethics* of a covert compulsory program supposedly promotes values such as liberty and autonomy. What an incredible distortion of the meaning of these words!

It's no surprise that the science shows that it's more effective to be covert. The covert form of abuse is much more dangerous because it can go so much further before people realize what's happening.

Observing the continual public health justification, *for the greater good*, we can expect to see more of this covert violation of consent in ongoing campaigns, including biotechnology and transhumanism.

CHAPTER 8

WHERE IS IT GOING?

The Science of Compliance

The disordered moral code of compliance is not just a tool of abusers and tyrants. It's also part of the New Normal brand of scientism.

The science of behavior control has been around for a long time. The term compliance is popping up more in articles and studies, specifically around the topic of "vaccine hesitancy." We will explore that in this chapter as well as what we can learn from those who were the least compliant with the abusive measures.

The science of compliance ought to be concerning to all of us, whether we've taken, or believe in, the experimental injectables or not. These tactics of coerced compliance won't just be limited to the COVID *plandemic* or the uptake of pharmaceutical products.

Coerced compliance can be used for any number of social control agendas, such as the "net zero carbon footprint" campaign. Some credit card companies are already tracking our estimated carbon emissions through our consumer habits. Airlines are also starting to include the carbon score on plane tickets to desensitize us to this agenda.

It may not sound alarming at first glance, but when we contemplate where this is going, we must take into consideration that humans exhale carbon dioxide. If the goal is "net zero" carbon, how long before governments and corporations start limiting our right to travel, make certain purchases, and even *breathe*?

Could it be that's why euthanasia programs are increasing around the world? How long before we start seeing marketing slogans asking us to *do our part* to make the planet healthier and cleaner? Call Medical Assistance in Dying (MAiD)? If that sounds like a far stretch, just consider all the things you never thought would be possible before 2020 and remember that abuse always escalates and public health campaigns are marketed *for the greater good*.

As we've explored earlier in this book, the goal of every abuser is compliance, and that's where the state of captivity leads the target.

People who have experienced the trauma of interpersonal abuse and healed to a certain degree usually feel alarmed by the pressure for compliance. We don't like a hard sell. This is because we were overtly forced or covertly coerced into doing things that weren't okay, things that violated our physical, psychological, or spiritual boundaries and led to harm.

It was shocking, but not surprising, to see the connections being drawn in the recent years to link trauma survivors with the shame of non-compliance, specifically regarding "vaccine hesitancy" and other public "health" measures.

The Guardian published a 2022 article called "Covid vaccine hesitancy could be linked to childhood trauma, research finds: With almost ten percent of the UK population unvaccinated, Public Health Wales surveys effects of early harm."[41]

The measures of the study are stated: nine different adverse childhood experiences, low trust in the National Health Service's COVID-19 information, supporting the removal of social distancing and mandatory face coverings, breaking COVID-19 restrictions, and vaccine hesitancy (rejection or uncertainty about vaccination).[42]

The study is titled on the Public Health Wales website as, "Coronavirus vaccine hesitancy linked to childhood trauma." It says that researchers are calling for support to "build trust in those affected."

> Reluctance or refusal to get vaccinated against Coronavirus infection (vaccine hesitancy), may be linked to traumatic events in childhood, such as neglect, domestic violence or substance misuse in the family home, suggests research funded by Public Health Wales and published in the BMJ Open.
>
> Research conducted with adults in Wales identified that vaccine hesitancy was three times higher among people who had experienced four or more types of childhood trauma than it was among those who hadn't experienced any.[43]

The main objective for this study listed in the medical journal *BMJ Open* reads:

> Adverse childhood experiences (ACEs) can affect life-course health and well-being, including risk-taking behaviour and trust. This study explored associations between ACEs and trust in health information on COVID-19, attitudes towards and compliance with COVID-19 restrictions and vaccine hesitancy.[44]

The study insinuates that not wanting to take the jab and non-compliance with the other (abusive) COVID measures are examples of the "risk-taking behaviors" of trauma survivors. It's ironic because it turns out we were right to recognize the risk-taking behavior of *receiving* the experimental injections as well as the harms of forced isolation and wearing a petri dish over our breathing holes.

The objective of the study also refers to the trust wound caused by childhood trauma. From my perspective, this study aims to *exploit* the trust wound of trauma survivors for the goal of figuring out how to get this demographic to comply with public health measures and campaigns: "Those who suffer in childhood are also least likely to trust official NHS [National Health Service] coronavirus information, follow the rules of restrictions or wear masks during the pandemic, public health experts found."[45]

No kidding. Our childhood traumas—and our active work on healing from those—gave some of us the discernment to recognize the red flags of abuse, coercion, authoritarianism, and manipulation. For many of us, childhood was like immersion training for these times.

It's fascinating that the higher the ACE score, the greater the mistrust for the public health campaign and the greater the awareness of the violation of consent: "The results showed that the more trauma people had experienced in childhood, the more likely they were to mistrust NHS Covid-19 information, to feel unfairly restricted by the government and to support the end of mandatory face masks."[46]

From what I've noticed among abuse survivors, only the ones who are empowered by actively taking responsibility for their lives and healing process are able to see through the covert abuse at the global level.

However, I noticed an exception among some trauma survivors whose primary defense mechanism is to fight. They sensed the abuse by authority figures, which reminded them of childhood. Fighting can be necessary at times for survival, though it can also be confused with empowerment. Fighting is false empowerment and doesn't mean that people are healing, self-responsible, or even aware of their traumas. But fortunately for many of them, that instinct to fight may have saved their lives and health in this case.

Many childhood trauma survivors who are still looking for answers and empowerment *outside* themselves fell into the COVID campaign abuse. This can include people who are aware of abuse in general yet still stuck in victimhood, where the focus is entirely external—on what the abusers did—as well as those in denial about their childhood trauma. This is because they haven't done the inner work yet.

The same happens at the micro level. Many people watch and read a lot of content on narcissists and psychopaths, wanting to know everything about those personality types. After a lot of research, they will come to believe that they know all the red flags, and that may be true at the level of the conscious mind. Yet because they haven't done the inner healing work, they often continue to fall into abuse dynamics because the subconscious programming from unresolved trauma is driving their behavior.

High-five to the childhood trauma survivors who have worked on their own healing enough to develop the discernment and self-trust necessary to recognize and not comply with the lying, deceptive, coercive, and controlling government, private organizations, corporations, and media.

The Guardian article about the study gives the appearance of caring about supporting trauma survivors. It almost sounds like the *Guardian* editors *just want to help them do the right thing* and get vaccinated.

> Results here suggest such individuals may have more difficulty with compliance with public health control measures and consequently require additional support. This is important not only for the current pandemic but for other public health emergencies arising in the future.[47]

Energetic discernment reveals that the editors don't actually care about *supporting* trauma survivors. If they did, they would have studied how to help trauma survivors to heal and how people are being traumatized by the public "health" measures. Instead, they covertly—though openly—admit it's all about compliance for this and future campaigns.

I'm calling attention to this study because the social engineers are warning us that COVID compliance was a test run for future campaigns. They will push compliance again, but next time with more data gathered from the beta test of 2020–2022, which they will manipulate and distort in order to coerce people into doing what they're told.

They want us to believe that we can't decide what's right for us as sovereign individuals. They want us to outsource our power and discernment to their designated trusted sources. They want us to consent to the atrocities justified by public health by sacrificing our human rights *for the greater good.*

In other words, they will have much more data (ammunition) to use against us next time they try to extort our trust and gain our compliance. We must learn from the past if we want to create a better future for ourselves and the generations who otherwise may be born in a post-consent world.

The weaponized science of compliance

It's important to remember that these social engineering tests and agendas are not limited to plandemics. Compliance is the name of the game and it's the future the social engineers want for human beings. They aren't even hiding it, though they are disguising it as *for the greater good.*

The social engineers have promoted the word "compliance" in corporate and medical culture for decades, which is a form of desensitization or priming. It's become comfortable and familiar for people working in those environments who don't question the words being used and what they really mean.

A nurse told me that medical providers use the term "non-compliant" to refer to patients who don't do what they're told, and this started long before COVID. He was referring to obese patients with heart disease who were eating junk food and not exercising. Of course, those are poor decisions; but people are free to make unhealthy choices, too. Though it's interesting how seamless it was for medical professionals to transfer the term "non-compliant patient" to those who didn't want to comply with the COVID experiments.

Since 2020, many words are being distorted from their actual meaning and altered in the public lexicon. It's helpful to look at the definitions before the influence of *newspeak*, as George Orwell called it in his famous book, *1984*.

The Merriam-Webster Dictionary defines "compliance" as following:

> **1 a:** the act or process of complying to a desire, demand, proposal, or regimen or to coercion
>
> Patient *compliance* in completing the treatment regimens was excellent.
>
> —Georgia A. Chrousos

> **b:** conformity in fulfilling official requirements
>
> His actions were in *compliance* with state law.
>
> **2:** a disposition to yield to others
>
> **3:** the ability of an object to yield elastically when a force is applied: flexibility[48]

It's interesting that the very first definition of compliance contains the word *coercion*. Compliance is a common behavioral response to coercion. When you hear the word compliance, notice the coercive language and elements. Those are the red flags of covert abuse.

I've seen some alarming scientific studies in which the goal was compliance. One example that I cited in Chapter 3 was the 2020 Yale study on the fear-based emotional manipulation in the vaccine messaging, in which the primary objective stated was to get people to comply with taking the shots.

A therapist from my network who is well aware of what's happening around the world, and who also experienced this kind of covert abuse in her personal life, sent me a link to a 2021 memo addressed to the Biden administration called "A Trauma Informed Approach to Vaccine Fear." She was shocked that some world-renowned trauma experts, several of whom we both learned from, signed this memo.

The trauma experts signed on as part of their "supportive guidance to the Administration" to get vaccine-hesitant trauma survivors to get vaxxed. Here we find trauma survivors being targeted by coercion campaigns used to gain trust for compliance.

The pretext for this one is the same as the Wales study mentioned earlier in this chapter—*Why are trauma survivors not getting vaxxed like everyone else?*

> The following memo has been developed with input from an interdisciplinary team of community, clinical and academic thought leaders from the trauma healing field to offer supportive guidance to the Administration. To successfully address this challenge, we need to shift

> the fundamental question from *"What's wrong with these people?"* to *"What happened to them?"* While the reasons for vaccine fear are diverse, complex and bipartisan, we believe that individual and collective trauma is an underlying issue responsible for attitudes and beliefs in the vaccine fear-laden population.[49] (Emphasis in original.)

It sounds so compassionate to shift the question from "What's wrong with these people [who don't comply]?" to "What happened to them?"

Can you imagine going to a therapist for something unrelated only to find out that the therapist is trying to coerce you to participate in a medical experiment or submit to a medical procedure by using language to make you feel validated as a trauma survivor in order to get you to doubt your own values, inner authority, self-trust and discernment? Talk about betrayal!

In an abusive relationship, a covert abuser will study all the points of weakness, pain, or vulnerability in the target. The abuser will first validate the target's pain and struggle, extracting the trust of the target who may not have the discernment to recognize acts of perceived kindness.

The grooming of trust through the perceived validation and compassion is used against the target. The sophisticated (covert) abusers—the ones who are masters of deception—use this tactic, as well as their enablers who think they're doing the right thing, or who are too scared to speak up.

Most of the trauma experts who signed that memo are probably not abusers but enablers. Will they own any accountability for coercing trauma survivors who may have been harmed or killed by those shots?

The memo gaslights us about choice: "Because trauma survivors have had their autonomy taken away at crucial periods of development, physical and psychological *safety and choice* is critical in meaningfully engaging them and allaying valid fear."[50] (Emphasis added.)

Again, it *sounds* like showing compassion for trauma survivors by purporting to create safety and choice. But it's also an instruction manual for how to covertly manipulate trauma survivors into doing what you want them to do, by using the right words and speaking to their specific pain points in order to get their compliance, while making them believe that it's their choice. Would you consider that complicity with evil?

Autonomy, safety, and choice are three keywords used in that paragraph. Let's explore each of these to understand how this language is being distorted and weaponized against trauma survivors who have wounds in all of these areas. In other words, let's shine light on the gaslighting.

Autonomy: In many places around the world, people were coerced by their employer, their doctor, or their government to take these potentially dangerous experimental drugs or lose their job, access to medical care, or the ability to enter public spaces. Where was the element of autonomy and self-governance for those who prefer other forms of treatment and prevention of illness based on what they know is best for them? It's not autonomy if a person is forced or coerced into compliance with the threat of losing his livelihood or being segregated from society. Have we not learned that segregation is degrading, dehumanizing, and an abuse of human rights?

Safety: The marketing campaign of *safe and effective* for the experimental drugs with unknown outcomes didn't win the trust of many trauma survivors. Some of us already knew the kind of covert abuse that can be hidden behind empty words and promises when people want our compliance with their desires and demands because *they just want to protect us and keep us safe*. They said they were doing it because they love us and because they care, but they destroyed us in the process. We know better than to believe such empty words because we have developed discernment, which is the subtle skill of reading energy and subtext. Promises of safety are often recognized as a red flag by those of us who learned this lesson the hard way.

Choice: The absence of real choice was alarming in cases where people were being coerced under duress into taking these experimental drugs. It was traumatic even for those of us onlookers who were watching other people being coerced instead of given a choice of their own free will. Many of us have been in relationships, whether personal or professional, where we were coerced into doing something we weren't okay with, which ended up harming us in some way. Later the abuser always says, "Well it was your choice. I didn't force you." When someone is removing the element of authentic choice through pressure, threats, and duress, that's always a red flag of abuse and manipulation.

The memo mentions four specific kinds of collective traumas to consider in addressing vaccine fear: medical system trauma, pharmaceutical industry trauma, racial trauma, and government/political trauma. Let's unpack the unfortunate irony here.

Medical system trauma: It's true that many people had already been abused by doctors and the medical system. We were taught to outsource the authority over our health decisions, and we were conditioned to outsource our power of choice, to the medical system. The memo ironically cites that medical error is the number three cause of death, and that indeed is a *very* important fact to consider before agreeing to any recommendations from doctors (or therapists) who were trained in that same medical system. Clearly something is wrong if medical treatment is one of the top reasons why people die prematurely in America.

Pharmaceutical industry trauma: It's true that many people have been harmed by this industry. Wise people are aware that Big Pharma is a medical mafia and the only legal drug dealers, with a long track record of paying fines for their criminal activity of falsifying studies that led to harm and death. So of course we don't trust their products, for which they don't even accept liability in case of harm and death. We have also seen how these corporations try to hide and manipulate data to avoid accountability for decades. Specifically, the pharmaceutical companies and the U.S. Food and Drug Administration (FDA) tried to ensure that the documents on the COVID- vax studies would remain secret for seventy-five years! Thankfully in January 2022, a group of scientists and medical researchers sued the FDA under the Freedom of Information Act. A federal court in the Northern District of Texas ordered the expedited release of hundreds of thousands of pages of the documents.[51] Since then, author Naomi Wolf's team has worked tirelessly to expose the horrors of those documents, while the vax campaigners continue to act like nothing happened. Wolf said the Pfizer documents contain evidence of "the greatest crime against humanity in the history of our species."[52] Why should we trust these corporations?

Racial trauma: The pharma-medical industry has a long track record of targeting people of color in cases like the forty-year Tuskegee experiment, which denied medical treatment to hundreds of black Americans who had syphilis[53] and the WHO-sponsored tetanus vaccine's "accidental" contamination of anti-fertility drugs used on millions of women and girls of childbearing age in Kenya.[54] Another example was the forced sterilization of hundreds of thousands of indigenous natives in Peru.[55] The Peruvian Ministry of Health used this campaign as part of its National Reproductive Health and Family Planning Program. *Reproductive health* is an interesting euphemism for population control and eugenics.

Government/political trauma: The memo cites that public trust in the government is at an all-time low. I think we can all agree on that point, no matter where we fall on the political spectrum. Only 2 percent of people polled by Pew Research said that they trust the government in Washington, DC, to do what is right "just about always," and 21 percent "most of the time."[56] The memo also mentioned that mistrust in government is mirrored in the public health system. This is *healthy* mistrust when we see that public health isn't about health at all.

All four of the specific collective traumas named in the memo are true, though distorted for the purpose of the campaign for vax compliance.

Toward the end, the memo makes what is perhaps the most egregious statement of this entire abomination:

> Telling the truth helps rebuild lost trust, so acknowledging the systems level trauma that has impacted so many individuals, families, and communities is going to be a key first step to any effective strategy in addressing vaccine fear. Much like the Truth & Reconciliation process, it will be impossible to re-establish trust without these institutions taking ownership of past actions that have been traumatizing and followed with a compassionate

> and empathetic message that mistrust / fear around the vaccine makes total sense and is completely valid.[57]

Again, it *sounds* like validation. And, yes, it's true that, whether we are talking about the systems (collective) level or individual level of trauma, telling the truth is the only way to start rebuilding lost trust. However, *the entire vax campaign was built on lies and emotional manipulation* and we are *still* not having an honest public conversation about it. Therefore, trust cannot be restored there.

One might wonder who drafted and sponsored that memo and how did they get world-renowned trauma experts to sign it?

On the bright side, the social engineers are subtly confirming something very important, that trauma survivors—particularly those who are facing the truth and actively working to take responsibility for their lives and their healing—are developing an increasing and natural immunity to abuse and manipulation.

The post-trauma state of disconnection

Trauma happens when an overwhelmingly stressful situation takes place, usually involving a perceived life threat to oneself or someone else in proximity. A person's life could actually be in danger or the person's nervous system could perceive a life threat. Either way, the terror gets frozen in the nervous system when there's a lack of safe, social connection at the time of the trauma.

Without an empathic witness or community, the opportunity for our nervous system to process the experience in the moment is lost. Then it becomes stored in the body and subconscious. This is why some people develop post-trauma symptoms and others don't, even when they experience a similar trauma.

In the animal kingdom, when a gazelle narrowly escapes becoming a lion's breakfast, the gazelle immediately shakes its entire body to discharge that energy. Then it goes to the group of its species for close contact. That facilitates the process of co-regulation, allowing the frightened gazelle to regulate its nervous system through the connection and safety of others' nervous systems.

Here's what *doesn't* happen when the gazelle attempts to connect and co-regulate with others:

"Well, was it really a trauma? How do we define trauma?"

"That's just life. Everyone knows lions eat gazelles. Why do you think you're special because you got chased by a lion? My friend was chased by *two* lions, *twice* as big as that one and she's fine. So, what's your problem?"

"The problem is that you went off on your own. It's your fault and you deserved it because you didn't do what the rest of us do. Stay in your lane!"

"I don't care. That sounds like a personal problem. I haven't experienced it so I can't be sure it's true that lions eat gazelles. Maybe you made it all up. You've always been dramatic."

Gazelles don't have those conversations. We humans do.

Mammals instinctually know to huddle together and connect after one of the group experiences a stressful event. Gazelles don't get post-trauma because they're not usually alone after the traumatic event. Humans are often physically alone or psychologically isolated, surrounded by others who are oblivious or dismissive.

In the human world, we often don't have anyone there in the moment to co-regulate with us. In that case, the trauma can't be processed and released in the moment. The post-trauma effect is caused when the trauma is frozen, which creates the ongoing and pervasive feeling of being unsafe. For childhood trauma survivors, the unsafe feeling can last a lifetime when left untreated or mistreated. That also leads to the repetition of more traumas.

Yet this sense of being unsafe is often not part of the person's conscious awareness. It's experienced as an anxiety felt deep in the body and subconscious, which continues to exist in the background. It becomes so familiar that a person might think such a state is normal.

Feeling unsafe becomes a constant in the trauma survivor's life, which leads to other secondary effects of the post-trauma, such as anxiety, panic, depression, substance abuse, other addictions, dysautonomia, and abusive relationships.

The post-trauma can be avoided when the trauma survivor is comforted—in the moment—by the loving, compassionate physical presence of others who acknowledge the terrifying experience and provide a safe social container. The survivor's autonomic nervous system will experience this kind of connection as safety. As mammals, we need to be able to co-regulate with others in this way so the fear doesn't get frozen in the nervous system, and instead can be processed and released.

What if people don't have others they can connect with, who can acknowledge that they see it, too, and can empathize that it's scary? What happens if those we go to are dismissive, don't understand or recognize what happened and why it mattered, or gaslight and abuse us?

For most of us going through traumatic life experiences, there wasn't anyone there in the moment, or anybody who recognized the impact of the event when we sought connection. Worse yet, people might blame the survivor. As kids, a lot of us didn't have anyone to run to. Even if there were people around, they didn't listen or believe us.

We tried to speak up about it and we were told things like:

"That didn't happen."

"Uncle Johnny would never do that."

"It's just your imagination."

"Stop spreading lies."

"So what, that's just life."

"Get over it. I did when it happened to me."

"Well I don't think anything happened to me!"

In the early 2020s, the isolation and fear bombardment were so intense in society that most people didn't have anyone to connect with. This was perhaps even more devastating for those of us who saw through the manipulation and abuse, feeling alone in that reality while others didn't see it, which reminded us of unresolved childhood trauma.

The experience of co-regulation between nervous systems is balancing and healing. Yet this depends on whether the empathic witness and survivor are able to connect without engaging each other's defensive reactions of fight, flight, freeze, and fawn.

During the COVID years, we were told not to touch or even be in close proximity with others. When the face masks were introduced and mandated (after we were first told that they don't work), eye contact also disappeared. There was fear caused by the sight of the mask. Part of the face was covered, which the nervous system would normally read for cues of safety or threat. That instinctually made people look away from others in order to feel safe.

If we want to experience the sense of safety created through social connection and co-regulation, we have to actively seek out people on the same page, with whom we can share eye contact, compassion, physical proximity, and in some cases physical touch. However, this only works when we are in relaxed states, and not in defense mode.

I also saw this happen with young children when I went to the grocery store during that time. When I wasn't wearing a mask, I smiled at little kids to offer them a friendly respite from the scary, cold, empty world of masked, fearful people. Every now and then I would get a smile back. But most of the time the kids instantly looked away. I became concerned about where this was headed for the future of our species.

What about the children who were emotionally, mentally, neurologically, and spiritually harmed during those traumatic years? Will they ever be able to experience healthy human connection or will their nervous systems continue to remember the feeling of disconnection triggered by others in physical proximity?

The COVID trauma happened during key developmental stages of the formation of children's brains and nervous systems. A US study showed a 20 percent decrease in the IQ of children during the lockdowns, which reduced their verbal, motor, and cognitive performance.[58] Can such damages be reversed? We don't know yet because this social experiment was never done before in human history.

Many people, including most trauma and abuse experts, still don't recognize the gravity of the collective and individual traumas that have been taking place. These fields seem to be more focused on gaining compliance than trauma healing. That's surreal, yet it also makes sense, given the covert nature of the abuse that's been happening around the world and the fact that mental health practitioners are not trained to recognize it. In fact, some of their training could be *hindering* their perspective, leaving their clients feeling more alone, traumatized, and misunderstood.

Many therapists are conditioned to believe and teach their clients that there's no such thing as good and evil. No wonder they couldn't see the evil behind what was happening.

The greatest trick the devil ever pulled was convincing us that he doesn't exist.

Of course there is nuance in life. Good people can sometimes do bad things, and bad people can sometimes do good things, yet to dismiss the existence of evil is dangerous.

When the truth comes out

Truth is being scrubbed from the internet and cast into the bin of censorship casualties in "the war on misinformation," which is really just a euphemism for anything that questions the Official Narrative.

For anyone who needs a reminder, *the good guys in history were never the ones censoring information*. As we explored in Chapter 1, abusers and tyrants always control the information in order to control the perception of reality in their favor.

The truth about the lack of safety and efficacy of the experimental shots, as well as the other harmful and ineffective public health measures, has been seeping out of the wounds of society after years of propaganda bombardment. However, most people are still in denial.

Like most survivors of abusive relationships, we may never find out the whole truth. If we want to liberate ourselves and heal, we ought to ask ourselves how much longer will we wait for external validation of the truth?

Unfortunately, abuse victims rarely get the truth, justice, or closure from their abusers. That's why most people never actually heal. They get stuck there and don't know how to move forward.

We might never know for sure how many millions of people were harmed by these irresponsible and *evil* public health campaigns. We might not ever know the names of all the puppet masters. We might not ever know what this phenomenon called COVID really was.

The majority of abuse survivors get stuck in the emotional attachment of wanting closure from the abusers and justice so they can move forward into the healing stages. Of the thousands of stories I've heard over the years, there were only a few where survivors got justice in legal or social systems.

Ideally, in a social system like a family, the rest of the family could stand with the victim and call the abuser(s) out for what they did. There could be a reckoning of the truth and that would be very relieving for the victim. But this rarely happens. It's usually the enablers who defend the abuser(s) and maintain the abusive system.

Abusers rarely admit what they did, and if they do confess little bits of the truth (acts of perceived kindness), it's only to extort your trust once again so they can continue abusing you. This is not the way to rebuild lost trust.

The corporations and institutions have never openly addressed the results from this mass medical experiment. One might wonder if they wanted the vax-trial data sealed in secrecy for seventy-five years so that everyone alive now would be dead by then. No one would be left to make claims for the truth or restitution. By then, history would have been re-written, like so many other distortions we were taught in school to be true.

An abuse victim tends to wake up after a particular event pierces her denial. She then begins to process what happened and name it as abuse. At some point, she will naturally begin to reflect upon her history, including that relationship and others. Once she starts identifying the abuse playbook, and recognizes how abusers all use the same tactics, she begins to see the patterns as if they were highlighted upon the fabric of reality. Once she sees these patterns, she can't unsee them. Even though she may never get concrete proof, or the truth from the abusers, her brain becomes more adept at the pattern recognition of manipulation.

Likewise, more people have awakened to the disruptive truth during the COVID plandemic when their denial was pierced. As they began to process the shock of what happened, and name it as abuse, many people naturally began to reflect upon history, wondering how many times they were deceived and abused without realizing. This is why many people are starting to take another look at events that happened in the past. They're beginning to see, in a new light, things they didn't question before.

While we may never know the full truth of what happened during the COVID plandemic, and many other things that happened in our world—such as wars, "pandemics," mass tragedy events, scandals, free energy, weather modification, or the deaths of JFK, MLK, and Jeffrey Epstein—we are certainly asking more questions. When we are dismissed, devalued, ostracized, smeared and shamed simply for asking questions, we recognize this as either a distraction tactic used by those who have something to hide or the defensiveness of those who are invested in the fantasy that they want to believe about their country, their politicians, their local authorities, their justice system, and the leaders of their religious institution or other identity group.

Several years ago, I was waiting in the checkout line at an organic shop in Mexico when I overheard a table of expats—Americans and Canadians—talking about a documentary called "Loose Change," which asks very relevant questions about what happened on the morning of September 11, 2001. One of the expats got really upset and said loudly, "No, I won't watch it because I can't live in a world in which that's true."

I believe denial is a force stronger than gravity. It takes much energy to overcome it. Yet once we see how easily the entire world was taken over by the manipulation in the COVID narrative, like any awakening abuse victim, we start to acknowledge that it couldn't have been the first time. The COVID plandemic was just the first time many of us *realized* we were being lied to and abused.

In retrospect, there are eerily similar patterns left in the footprints of history, as well as in current events. I was in a trauma training last year where a guest speaker, a licensed psychologist, was speaking about climate change being one of the main causes of anxiety nowadays. Referencing the American Psychological Association's Climate Change Psychology Advisory Group, she stated that the most important thing is to believe climate scientists. This is from the same playbook as "listen to the COVID experts and don't do your own research or think for yourself because the experts know best." Propaganda is woven into the institution of psychology for the purpose of promoting behavioral modification.

We are very likely never going to get the proof we seek or the whole truth from the abusers, past and present. The only way to start healing from abusive relationships and situations is to stop outsourcing our power by wanting the perpetrators to admit what they did, or are doing. That attachment can keep an abuse target frozen in time, unable to move forward, stuck in the powerlessness of victimhood and continuing to repeat more of the past.

Even if all the truth were to be exposed, it's also likely that much of society continues to act as enablers, maintaining the status quo and pretending nothing happened. Trying to wake everyone up is not where we will find our power to move forward.

It would be awesome if international lawyers and judges could pursue justice and accountability for the crimes committed against humanity. In an ideal world that would happen. But in our world, most people are compromised by their own distorted desires and our justice systems are incredibly corrupt. How long will it take for justice to take place? Five years? Ten? Twenty? Fifty?

Wise people—many of whom are recovering abuse survivors—are able to recognize that there can be no trust where there is no *truth, the whole truth, and nothing but the truth*. How can we ever trust these corporations and institutions (as well as those who are enabling them) when they're *still* gaslighting us?

In my experience, when people don't take accountability for what they did, it means they don't believe they did anything wrong, and they'll likely do it again. This unfortunately includes the enablers. If they can't face the truth and admit what they enabled, then go through an internal reckoning process about the decisions they made, they will likely do it again.

Many people regret taking the experimental drugs and refuse to take more now. People have told me that they don't know why they got jabbed and went along with it. Some cited family weddings. Others didn't know how to provide for their families without their job. Some were afraid to submit exemption requests for fear of social ostracism and retaliation.

I've looked into the teary, remorseful eyes of parents who had their kids injected because they didn't want them to be isolated any longer from peers and family. I have compassion for people who were coerced into it thinking they were doing the best thing they could.

Many of us know people who have been harmed or killed after getting the shots.[59] We're continually reading about cases of healthy and fit young people, such as top athletes, collapsing, dying suddenly, or having sudden heart and blood issues among other tragedies.[60]

Unfortunately, many people only stopped complying because they are no longer being threatened and coerced to do so. These people are still subscribed to the Official Narrative, which means they are but one fear campaign away from being terrified right back into compliance and enabling the abuse.

When you're the only one in your social circle who sees through the agenda of compliance, while everyone else is acting like nothing happened, you can start to doubt yourself from all the group-think and crazymaking.

That's when it's a good time to remind yourself of Krishnamurti's famous statement: "It's no measure of health to be well adjusted to a profoundly sick society."

CHAPTER 9

WHERE ARE WE NOW?

In Between Worlds

The past got us to where we are now. It will not get us to where we want to be, if we want to create a different world than the one we are currently living in, which is clearly *not* working.

After the intense stresses of the early 2020s, we are now in a strange limbo state.

Many people are saying that nothing makes sense anymore—that something is wrong, but they don't know what it is. Others express feeling like everyone is dead inside. I also hear people saying that their perception of time is very weird and *life feels surreal.*

The strangeness of these feelings, which can be difficult to name and describe, is quite similar to the unsettling time after a person leaves an abusive relationship or family system, after divorce, the loss of a job or home, the death of a loved one, an injury or illness, or even after a war. People often go through a void in which they don't know what to do with themselves or their life.

In these in-between spaces, we are no longer in the old world and identity, yet also not fully in the new. So where are we?

In this chapter, we'll explore our present predicament as individuals and society in order to inspire the hope that not all is lost. We can use the hidden potential in our current liminal experiences for growth, wisdom, and evolution.

We have been through tremendous experiences so far this decade, and that trend will likely continue. *What matters is what we do with it.*

Thresholds of transformation

A transitional state or place is referred to as a liminal space. When a sense of loss or massive change happens, it catapults us into these strange in-between spaces and places. It can feel even more overwhelming when we didn't want those changes to happen and we wish we could go back to how things were. This is the crux after trauma.

These kinds of experiences have always been part of human life. Most people have suffered multiple unexpected losses since 2020. All of us lost something, some a lot more than others.

Early on, people lost jobs and businesses that weren't baptized as "essential" by public health officials. Most people lost the ability to see others during the social distancing. Some lost income and educational opportunities. Many lost loved ones, whether through death or unreconcilable differences in the perception of reality. Some lost their self-respect when they took the jab even though they didn't want to just so they could see loved ones, especially those in care homes or at a distance requiring travel. Some lost their health to the bioweapons and social isolation. Some lost the in-person support of their doctors, therapists, and other practitioners who closed their doors and shifted to telehealth. Some chose to leave everything behind and move to new states or countries to escape the tyranny or trade in a bigger threat for a smaller one.

In Part Two of this book, we'll explore ways of processing and integrating the loss and trauma in order to regenerate resilience for thriving as liberated souls. But first it's important to understand the nature of the in-between process as we are moving through the heavy fog in this unfamiliar forest of liminality.

Regardless of the personal impact of the losses incurred, we all lost a degree of illusion and certainty. None of us believed the entire world could lock down in a matter of weeks, changing human life so drastically in such a short period of time. No matter what perspective we have about what was happening, what we all have in common is that our reality has been shattered and it will never be like it was before 2020.

As if in suspended animation, many are wondering when they will return to a normal living state. The past is frozen in our bodies and local energy fields as well as in the collective consciousness. This leaves things feeling unsettling, uncertain, and surreal. The clock is ticking, the calendar is progressing, but where are we?

We are being challenged to adapt to a rapidly changing world as we are walking through these liminal spaces as individuals and society.

Liminal comes from the Latin word meaning the point at which a physiological or psychological effect begins to be produced. It's often used to describe a threshold or transitionary period—a state of transition.

Liminal spaces refer to the transitional phases, places or states of being that exist between one reality and another. These spaces are known for ambiguity, disorientation, and a sense of possibility.

A physical liminal space could be a doorway, hallway, or airport. It could also represent the transition between the old world and the new.

An emotional or psychological liminal space could be transitional phases of life like adolescence, grieving or recovery from trauma, a breakup, illness, or addiction. It could also be the space between having a massive perspective shift where a person is no longer who he was but not yet fully embodying the upgraded identity.

A metaphorical liminal space could be the inner conflict of indecision between making one decision vs. another, each of which will have a different path forward.

Social liminal spaces are periods of collective upheaval, such as the aftermath of wars, plandemics, natural disasters, or cultural shifts. It could also represent the time between an election and the inauguration of a new president or prime minister. Liminality involves periods of transition and uncertainty accompanying personal or collective crises.

Surely there have been many social experiences of liminality in human history, both globally and locally. We are living in perhaps one of the most interesting ones. Artists, writers, and thought leaders have always explored liminality as fertile ground for innovation, discovery, and creativity.

After World War I and the so-called Spanish flu pandemic, society experienced a profound sense of liminality. It was a time of personal and collective disorientation, disillusionment, grieving, and uncertainty, with parallels to the feelings and experiences that many of us face today.

The 1920s were marked by the dissolution of order and a loss of faith in traditional structures—political, religious, social, and financial—which failed to prevent the devastation. Of course, knowing what we know now, it's likely that the social engineering behind those very institutions *contributed* to the events that occurred. The economic boom of the decade ended in the Great Depression.

In the aftermath of the atrocities experienced in the postwar and post-pandemic period, people surely struggled to make sense of what happened and grieve what had been lost, while grappling with the uncertainty of what could emerge afterward. Understandably, most people likely preferred not to face it and really unpack what happened, instead relegating those memories to the pit of oblivion.

The same thing often happens after experiences involving massive personal loss. It's incredibly painful, which is why it's tempting to suppress it and avoid dealing with it. Sometimes the survivor will summon the courage to introspect and dig deeper into her personal healing and growth, later emerging from the liminal space with a renewed sense of resilience, identity, meaning, joy, and purpose.

It's interesting to notice what happened in the artistic and cultural responses that emerged in the 1920s, which can offer us some valuable insight into our time. The Roaring Twenties were a wild and booming period of economic prosperity and modernity in America. It was a bold break from old traditions and order.

The Jazz Age and more risqué forms of dancing became popular, perhaps as people wanted to forget about the morbid and oppressive events that had taken place during the war. A period of cultural liberation and musical experimentation started, perhaps reflecting a desire to embrace life more in the face of mortality, disempowerment, and uncertainty. The trauma was emerging into expression through art.

Surrealism as an artistic movement emerged in Europe directly from the liminal space of the early 1920s, emphasizing the irrational and unconscious as tools for navigating a fractured reality. Existentialists were also exploring themes of meaning, alienation, and purpose while trying to make sense of a chaotic world. Creativity was booming in certain pockets of society.

Mass production and consumerism also boomed, allowing America's middle class more access to the new technological developments. Celebrities and other cultural heroes became the focal point of idealization among a society eager to replace the traumatic memories with a stimulating fantasy.

In the 1920s, the personal and collective grief was bypassed. Denial is a survival mechanism that can help in the short-term, yet inevitably becomes maladaptive in the long run, which is exactly how history keeps repeating itself.

Likewise, in the 2020s, we are now navigating the liminal spaces between the pre-2020 world and the new world. We're all trying to make sense of things. Surely some nefarious players would like to create a New World Order, as they've so frequently warned us for decades. They want us to "reimagine" that world with them. In fact, they can't do it without us.

If we sleepwalk through the liminality—confused, lost, dissociated, and drifting without direction into idealization, technological developments, rescue fantasies, and consumerism—we could easily fall into the trap laid out for us. Alternatively, we can make different choices, instead navigating the liminality consciously and with purpose.

The key to that door opening to prosperity is creativity and responsibility. And, as explored earlier in this book, when we are in the state of captivity, we are disempowered and locked out of higher states of consciousness such as insight, intuition, imagination, and creativity.

Many people are barely hanging on. They feel overwhelming anxiety and uncertainty, as well as the deep confusion that comes with feeling caught between the pre-2020 "normal" and the unknown future. Our old systems and structures have been crumbling at the seams, yet new ones have not fully formed. People are questioning how much power we have in these matters or if we are merely drifting in a sea of chaos.

While nothing will ever be like it was before 2020, and it's true that after trauma we can never go back to how things were before, that doesn't have to be a bad thing. We don't have to create the new world based on what the global mafia want. We have the option of recognizing this liminal space as the incredibly fertile ground it is for personal transformation and creating the kind of world that we *actually* want to live in.

As we navigate the aftermath of the plandemic, drifting into the potential for multiple wars as well as rapidly accelerating technological developments, unsustainable national debt, and inflation, we are also seeing increasing political and ideological polarization, economic instability, and an epidemic of mental illness.

While the liminality can be deeply uncomfortable, it is also true that these are times of potentiality. When we realize and accept that our existing paradigms aren't working any more, that shift in perspective offers the possibility of growth, renewal, and regeneration. It's an invitation for reflection and inspiration—a calling to evolve through new ways of thinking, healing, living, being, and connecting with ourselves and one another.

Like in the 1920s, in the 2020s the liminality serves as a space where trauma can be repurposed through art. With the gift of retrospect and learning from what happened before, we can be more intentional this time.

We are yet again living in times of crumbling old systems, though now as a *much* more globalized world with larger ripple waves. This is shaking our sense of foundation and security, both individually and collectively. Navigating the liminality requires leaning into the physical, emotional, mental, and spiritual existential void of uncertainty.

Art offers us the unique ability to access parts of ourselves that we might not otherwise be able to contact verbally or intellectually. It gives us permission to imagine, visualize, and express feelings and possibilities that transcend our current uncertainties, fears, limitations, and restraints. Art can travel places that words cannot go.

Art provides a metaphorical space where we can express complex emotions and confront subconscious fears in a way that's perhaps less overwhelming or threatening. Art is a vehicle for initiating the processing of grief and trauma at the individual and collective levels. It's also a way to create new clarity from chaos.

We can artistically re-frame the narrative about the changes taking place in our world by creating a new dialogue between the past, present, and future. Art can play a vital role in allowing us to feel, express, observe, and process as we move through the liminality toward liberation and the creation of greater wellbeing for ourselves as individuals and the human race.

Trying to make sense of a fractured world

I majored in Spanish in college, and the curriculum included literature and art as well as the language. In one of the advanced semesters, I took a class on surrealism. I didn't really understand it until I had the gift of retrospect from the post-2020 world. Now it's starting to make more sense.

Our professor toured us through the life and works of famous surrealists, such as Salvador Dalí and Luis Buñuel. We watched an absurd short film called *Un Chien Andalou* (1929) by Dalí and Buñuel, which left a strong mark on my memory. We discussed themes like whether Dalí's melting clocks in the dreamlike landscape of *The Persistence of Memory* (1931) offer more insight than merely being considered the work of a mad man.

A few years ago, when I heard people talking about how surreal life feels nowadays, I remembered that class and did some reflecting. I discovered that there is a connection between the surrealist movement and trauma that can help us to understand more about the times we are living in, exactly one hundred years later.

The unprecedented horrors of the Great War and so-called Spanish flu pandemic influenced many artists and thought leaders of the 1920s to reject the accepted societal values and explore new ways of understanding the human experience. Perhaps in an attempt to understand how something so disturbing could have happened, they set out to create meaning from the disorder and loss.

The surrealist movement was a rebellion against the rationalism and materialism that was believed to have led to the Great War. The widespread suffering and existential crises influenced the cultural and artistic milieu from which surrealism emerged. *Art was used to try to make sense of the world.*

Many artists were sent to the frontlines during that time. There are some uncanny parallels of war, the plandemic, and political upheavals occurring then and now. Though in the 2020s, it seems the order is reversed, and the kinetic wars are coming after the plandemic.

The Spanish flu pandemic came right on the heels of the war and was mostly overshadowed by it. Several influential artists and writers died of illness, though direct artistic representations of the Spanish flu were rare. This scarcity is likely due to the overwhelming desire to move forward afterward, much as we see nowadays. As terrifying as war is, perhaps it was easier to name than the invisible threat of disease.

Was the Spanish flu a pandemic or plandemic? If you've seen any of the old newspaper photos circulating the internet since 2020, from 100 years before during the so-called Spanish flu, you may have been as shocked as me to see almost identical propaganda. There were newspaper clippings of very similar mask mandates with fear bombardment and intimidation, as well as smear campaigns against the "mask slackers". There were photos of flyers created by activists holding anti-mask meetings and warning people against vaccines. There's also the famous photo of the frontline workers in their SOS motor cars wearing masks. In the background, a tightly gathered, and seemingly unafraid, group of elite men in suits were standing there unmasked, quietly directing the operation.

A century later, the playbook of reality distortion and manipulation appears eerily similar. It's also interesting that there's speculation that much of the illness back then was caused by chemical warfare from World War I, and most deaths due to bacterial pneumonia, which can happen from wearing masks. Likewise, in 2020, there was speculation of various toxins that could have caused people to get sick before the masking and injections began. The effects of the trauma caused by the shock, confusion and terror that people experienced are also likely to leave similar consequences on modern society and individuals, as it did 100 years ago.

André Breton was a medical student during World War I where he served in the medical corps. He also worked in neuropsychiatric wards treating soldiers who suffered from shell shock, which we now call post-traumatic stress disorder (PTSD). Breton's first-hand wartime experiences with traumatized soldiers played a pivotal role in shaping the philosophical and creative foundations of surrealism. After the war, he re-directed his exploration from medicine and science to art, literature, and creativity, which allowed him access to the realm beyond the conscious mind.

Breton and other surrealists had direct experience with the atrocities of the war. This caused them to view trauma as a force of darkness that shatters conventional realities and exposes the deeper—and darker—truths about humanity. Their work was an attempt to confront the pervasive sense of loss and instability that they sensed within themselves and in society. Then, like now, there were probably few people talking about it.

Art can be a potent tool for catalyzing the healing process of psychological and spiritual wounds. It's also helpful for understanding and transmitting the hidden aspects of human experience, especially those that are felt deeply yet are difficult to explain in thoughts or words.

The surrealist movement became known for themes like liberating the mind, using the juxtaposition of the ordinary and the extraordinary, exploring dreams and the unconscious, as well as political and social rebellion.

One could interpret the surrealist movement as an artistic response to the insanities of modern life, namely the devastation and chaos of the early twentieth century. The artists and writers sought to create new meaning in a fractured world by using the imagination as a tool for healing, exploration, and resistance to oppression.

While the surrealists aimed for freedom of thought, they also got caught up in reactionary political ideologies as well as Freudianism, which heavily influenced surrealism and led to a fracturing within the movement. Trauma often leads to reactive stances in an attempt to create safety and meaning.

Dalí was one of the few who initially wanted art to remain apolitical, which caused discord with other surrealists. When Francisco Franco won the civil war in his home country of Spain, Dalí endorsed the new ruler and the Spanish fascists, perhaps because he wanted to maintain his property and status in his homeland. He was then kicked out of the surrealist movement.

The surrealists mostly aligned with the ideologies of communism and anarchism. They criticized the bourgeois norms and systems, which the surrealists saw as oppressive. They'd also mock the hypocrisies of the bourgeois class. However, they didn't see how communism is also oppressive and how its popularity as a form of rebellion was a reactionary stance to the overt fascism taking over parts of Europe. It's interesting that we see similar patterns today.

The surrealist movement became a threat to the Nazis who wanted to suppress intellectual resistance and liberation. The Nazis categorized surrealism (as well as other modernist and avant-garde movements) as degenerate art, trying to eliminate anything that could inspire intellectual dissent in any form. Several of the surrealists spent time as prisoners in concentration camps.

In the late 1930s, André Breton and his wife Jaqueline Lamba, also a surrealist artist, were targeted by the Nazis. Along with many other prominent artists and writers, they connected with the Emergency Rescue Committee, which helped them to escape southern France after the occupation and board a ship heading to Martinique, eventually arriving in America.

The persecution and exile experience during World War II forced the artists and intellectuals to face displacement as well as a loss of community, home, and culture. They were again searching for meaning in an unstable world. That affected their work and the overarching surrealist ideals.

Having been forced from their homeland as political refugees, they deepened their artistic exploration of themes like liminality, belonging and the human condition—the very themes that are affecting many of us today. Those who were persecuted for bravely standing up for the values of freedom, liberation, and defiance of oppression in the 2020s can relate to the experiences of the surrealists.

The COVID narrative and the justification of the irrational and abusive mandates were supposedly based on science and rationalism. This has left many people disillusioned with the established systems of materialism, science, and public health, questioning the social consensus that led to such atrocities.

The global mafia, who continue to come up with the script, propaganda, policies, and narratives have always made *rules for thee, but not for me*. We saw so many examples of tyrannical government officials exempting themselves from the rules they tried to force on We the People in the name of public health. Not even public shaming could stop them when they were caught on camera, which is much easier nowadays than it was in the 1920s. Nonetheless, they went on like nothing happened.

The bourgeoisie hasn't changed much in one hundred years, though it's interesting how the ideology of Marxism has been coming back around as a misleading solution to the problem. This time the identity politics are going beyond socioeconomic class, now including race and gender themes, contributing to the divide and conquer of We the People. The more we identify with groups, the more easily we are manipulated against one another.

By the 2020s, we had seen clear elements of neo-Marxism infiltrating our school systems, military, and culture in insidious ways that have contributed to the fragmenting of society, an increased sense of entitlement, and a loss of self-responsibility and meritocracy that is healthy for a thriving society where innovation and progress are incentivized.

These ideologies, while perhaps implemented from a desire for radical change in a society that has run amok with trauma, abuse, and chaos, have not led to *positive* change and instead have contributed to the social rot in our institutions and the collective consciousness, and in the shredding of the fabric of humanity.

Art has the power to transcend propaganda and psychological programming—though it can also be hijacked by infiltrators to serve the purpose of propaganda and psychological programming.

If we look below the surface of political reactionism, we can see the deeper truths in the surrealist movement about the failures of traditional systems, including the medical establishment and social hierarchies. This is why the surrealists sought refuge in the unconscious mind as a space of freedom, creativity, and rebellion against the oppressive forces of their time.

Yet the unconscious alone does not give us a full picture of the human being or the process for healing after such traumas and atrocities. We need to *make the unconscious conscious*, as Carl Gustav Jung said. Transcending the darkness also requires distilling clarity from chaos.

The works of surrealism create an emotionally provoking catharsis, encouraging viewers to question reality and confront their own subconscious fears and desires. Surrealism wasn't meant to be understood in a rational way with a traditional artistic sensibility. It was meant to catch by surprise and provoke the viewer to *feel* something viscerally. Perhaps this was an attempt at liberating souls from the inner prison and numbness of the state of captivity.

Taking into account their psychosocial environment at the time, these elements appear to confront what was frozen in the subconscious of individuals and society. The surrealists expressed the suppressed emotional burden of trauma, confusion, fear, and uncertainty that was *absenced* in a society of individuals unable to feel or talk about it because it was too scary and painful.

Reconnaissance of the terrain ahead

Avant-garde art, like surrealism, emerges during periods of historical upheaval, reflecting the societal tensions and inner dilemmas of individuals. It disrupts the status quo, critiquing the framework or assumptions that mass culture assumes or takes for granted. Those who push the edges of the collective consciousness and challenge the popular culture's worldview are often considered ideologically unacceptable by the establishment of the time.

In an 1825 essay, *The Artist, the Scientist and the Industrialist,* Benjamin Olinde Rodrigues called upon the moral obligation of artists to serve as the avant-garde of the people, leading the way to societal change.

Avant-garde comes from a military term that means advanced guard, a reconnaissance unit that scouts the terrain ahead of the rest of the army.

What will become the next controversial trend of avant-garde art, challenging the status quo and innovating new forms of expression about our world during the intensely stressful experiences of the 2020s?

What will it say about us and about the times in which we live nowadays, and how will it inspire positive change?

The avant-garde of our time will emerge from artists, writers and other creators—thought leaders—whose perspectives, creativity, and works challenge the consensus worldview and disrupt comfort zones, including those aligned with popular causes.

I would bet that the post-2020 avant-garde art becomes less about physical or visual objects and more about immersive, participatory experiences since so many people are now craving connection more than stuff.

There's a growing desire for shared human experiences in our fragmented world. A sense of deep human connection is what's missing. I believe the avant-garde art of our time will allow us to process trauma collectively through a living medium. It may involve the responsible integration of technology as well as a seeking of simplicity and harmony with nature amidst the ever-growing complexities of our worldly concerns.

In order to exit the cycle of insanity—doing the same thing and expecting different results—what we need is a way to process the individual and collective grief amidst the existential crises of our world, while being cautious where we place our trust and hope. We ought to be mindful of the social engineering influence that will try to infiltrate, corrupt, and distort any genuine grass-roots movements that emerge from the liminality of these times.

Liminality can be leveraged for creativity, positive innovations in technology, personal development, and culture. Art is one of our most potent vehicles for catalyzing the heavy energy that we've been carrying so we can emerge more liberated into a new way of living and being.

History repeats itself when we don't resolve the past

Europe was left in ruins after the wars, plandemic, and economic devastation of the first half of the 1900s. Most of the prominent artists sought refuge in America during the persecution of World War II, putting New York at the epicenter of the avant-garde.

The artistic trends shifted again in the postwar era, when abstract expressionism became the new symbol of freedom and individuality, which was also aligned with the values and worldview of the United States.

On the heels of World War II, the theme of existential anxiety came to the forefront with the shifting global order and the fears of nuclear annihilation during the growing tensions of the Cold War.

The art emerging during that time could be described as having a sense of urgency in the way that it evoked deep subconscious emotions while also aiming to create a universal, spiritual, or transcendent experience. The art was both responding to the global traumas and uncertainty as well as offering the hope of resilience and renewal. Of course, it was also influenced by the social engineering trends of that time.

In the post–World War II years, the tyranny went underground and became much more covert. The best place for evil to hide is under the cloak of humanitarianism and philanthropy. The United Nations was created ostensibly as a solution to the atrocities of the Holocaust and World War II.

The 1950s was a bizarre decade of post-liminality, flavored with themes of consumerism and idealization in the new American life. The Interstate highways were being constructed and fast-food chains began to explode with the car culture. Millions of American veterans received GI bill home loans with the promise of social mobility and other enticements to follow the suburban sprawl. They were expected to start families in the new world, producing the next generation of indoctrinated children.

Social engineering and indoctrination rolls from generation to generation. The underlying patterns are the same, while the messaging and cultural context shifts, much like we've seen in the plandemics and wars. It's all the same playbook—reality distortion, psychological and spiritual torture, intermittent acts of perceived kindness, fantasies presented as welcome escapism, and system dynamics—updated in cultural and situational circumstances.

The boom of American cars, advertising, music, and consumer culture was engineered to reprogram people after the trauma with happy, idealized memories, and fantasies. It was surely a lot easier to focus on an enticing life of convenience and distraction than to face the unresolved past or the present threat of nuclear annihilation. There was a mix of fantasy, hope, and fear.

Meanwhile, millions of children were trained to do duck-and-cover drills like Bert the Turtle. In the 1951 civil defense film *Duck and Cover*, American children were told, "We must be ready every day, all the time, to do the right thing if the atomic bomb explodes."[61] A catchy tune and various scenarios were simulated showing kids what to do when they're alone or without adults. Surely many kids had nightmares from those images, fearing isolation when the worst-case scenario happens. Hiding under desks or under a thin cloth from the nuclear threat and atomic fallout was an absurd illusion of safety juxtaposed with terror.

In 1950, only 10 percent of American households had a television. By 1959, 90 percent did.[62] This was an unprecedented shift in media and messaging. No longer just reading or hearing information, people began to receive transmissions and programming via imagery.

The Golden Age of Television and celebrity culture also came in the postwar era, giving people endless distraction and entertainment so they didn't have to think about the past. *We don't ask about war stories*. Instead people sat around the TV, where they were hypnotized, bonding over their favorite sitcoms showing them how to be the perfect 1950s family.

Ignoring trauma leads to cycles of suppression, depression, and violence, which creates more trauma. Narcissism skyrocketed with the baby boomer generation born in the postwar era. I believe that was due to the unprocessed trauma of their parents who understandably just wanted to move on after the wars, the plandemic, and the Great Depression, which had marked the first few decades of their lives. Surely, they wanted to save their kids from having to know what that was like. They unknowingly transferred their unresolved trauma to the kids, which was promoted by the social engineering of the idealized 1950s fantasy life, alternated with the torture of the fear of nuclear annihilation. Once again, we see the socially engineered abuse cycle of idealization and devaluation, calm and chaos. This keeps people in a perpetual state of insecurity and instability.

The unsustainable collective fantasy of that so-called Golden Age brought a false sense of safety and a bypassing of the trauma. It certainly wasn't a "golden age" for everyone, as groups of people were still being segregated and discriminated against based on their skin color, gender and sexuality. It also wasn't golden for the poor. The idealization of the Golden Age was marketed to the privileged class in America, who had the illusion of freedom. It didn't take long for the flight into fantasy of the 1950s to begin bursting at the seams.

The 1960s was a decade of more trauma-based mind control with multiple famous assassinations of cultural heroes televised along with political upheavals, civil rights movements and riots, police brutality, counterculture, spiritual awakening throttled by escapism through drug abuse and promiscuity disguised as "free love" or "sexual liberation", and a war in Vietnam that no one wanted to fight. Yet another generation of youngsters got thrown into war trauma.

The space race offered a fantasy and escape from the social turmoil and unprocessed shock and trauma, topping off the end of the decade with a Stanley Kubrick-esque moon landing spectacle on film. It's striking that the only times humans reportedly traveled beyond the Van Allen radiation belt into deep space, occurred at the end of one of the most psychologically fragmented decades in modern history—the 1960s. That era followed the "Golden Age" illusion of the decade of the 1950s, which was marked by the trauma of the post-war anxiety and nuclear dread. And that decade followed a succession of global crises:

two world wars, the Great Depression and a previous pandemic—all largely unprocessed in the collective psyche.

Now in the afterglow of the COVID era awakening, do you also have questions about whether humans really went to the moon? I'm not suggesting everyone was "in on it." Likewise, I doubt that most of the world's leaders who deployed the top-down policies locally were *consciously* participating in the COVID narrative. I think most of them were manipulated by the social engineering to react in predictable ways based on their own disordered desires and unresolved trauma, as well as the subconscious distortions impacting their perception of reality and the phenomenon of group think—much like these same factors can affect the rest of us.

We lived through a moment when nearly the entire world was pulled into a shared belief: that COVID was so terrifying, it required our total obedience, and that the only truth was the one being broadcasted. But what unfolded was not what we were told. And now, rather than speaking openly about what happened, most of society is pretending that it didn't happen.

This collective silence doesn't dissolve the distortion. It *buries* it. And what is buried doesn't disappear. It becomes inheritance, ossified into belief structures. When future generations look back, they won't know what really happened. They'll be told the Official Story, and they'll probably believe it because there will be nothing else in the history books or on the digital record. This is how emotional residue, distortion and unprocessed trauma silently pass from one generation to the next. Unspoken distortion becomes unexamined inheritance.

Belief isn't just thought; It's architecture. Most of what we believe, we didn't choose. We inherited it—from culture, family, religion, and trauma. These beliefs form the invisible scaffolding of how we see the world, like an unseen frame holding up what we call "reality." It feels heavy because we are carrying the weight of the distortions we inherited. And at some level we sense the tension between what we've been taught to believe and what actually resonates.

The world feels heavier to each new generation because our species is outgrowing our inherited scaffolding. We aren't just watching the collapse of systems in our world. We are feeling the collapse of the invisible inner scaffolding—the beliefs that shaped those systems and once held it all together. And while that collapse may feel disorienting, it's actually an invitation.

Rather than debate scientific or observational details about the Apollo missions, my questioning is based on my area of focus—the generational trauma and narrative imprinting operating in the background—and why re-examining those events from a new perspective could be key to interrupting the repetitive patterns that are likely to recur in our time.

Earlier in this book, we explored how trauma fragments the self, creating dissociation, memory gaps and susceptibility to suggestion. In states of brain fog, humans are more vulnerable to manipulation, not because we are weak, but because the body-mind is overwhelmed.

In the 1960s, this vulnerability was compounded by the rapid rise of pharmaceuticals—tranquilizers and other psychotropic drugs—that subtly alter perception and behavior. Many American men numbed themselves with work routines and alcohol. Many housewives, prescribed psychiatric drugs, moved through their days while exposed to a constant stream of subliminal messages from the TV playing in the background. People were understandably trying to cope, to soothe, to not feel what hadn't yet been named.

Meanwhile psychologists began transforming advertising into a behavioral science by studying consumer behavior in focus groups. No longer responding to what people wanted, advertising began strategically shaping future desires through feedback loops and image-based entrainment for billboards and television.

The counterculture appeared to be a separate current—but it too was touched by distortion. What began as an awakening of collective consciousness, inspired by psychedelics and Eastern wisdom traditions, was mostly diverted by distorted human desires and co-opted narratives. The introduction of the contraceptive pill coincided with the normalization of behaviors previously considered taboo—some rooted in sovereignty and others in escapism.

Rebellion, when untethered from clarity, often leads to choosing the opposite pole of the same illusion. Both poles tend to be co-opted by empire. What the mainstream and counterculture had in common was an unconscious desire to leave the body, to avoid what was too painful to process. It was in many ways, a time of collective *flight*.

Given the pharmacological, psychological and cultural forces in motion, would most people have had a clear perception of reality in the 1960s? Or were they invisibly guided toward fantasy because it was too much to face the full weight of reality?

It was during that peak moment of cultural destabilization that Steward Brand, a Stanford-trained idealist and systems thinker, launched a campaign in 1966: *Why haven't we seen a photograph of the whole Earth yet?*[63] He made buttons and sold them at college campuses. He also sent them to scientists, engineers and policymakers at NASA. Perhaps he was just a guy with an interesting idea. Or maybe he was unknowingly influenced by forces in his environment to play a role that would forever alter human history.

Brand believed that such an image of the Earth could catalyze a planetary awakening—a shift from divisiveness to unity. Yet the planetary unification narrative is often a distortion. It tends to circle back to dependency on institutions and empire.

Brand's wish was fulfilled on Christmas Eve of 1968—at a time when many Americans were immersed in the dream-like holiday trance, another post-war socially-engineered fantasy. Simultaneously, the nation was reeling from the Vietnam war, civil unrest, and a string of devastating assassinations. Life must've felt incredibly surreal.

The Official Story goes like this: Apollo 8 was the first manned flight to leave Earth's orbit, reach the moon, circle it, and return. A U.S. telecommunications company launched a satellite a week ahead of time to ensure global audiences could tune into the broadcast. On that night, during the most-watched worldwide television event to date, the astronauts aboard Apollo 8 took turns reading the first 10 verses of the Book of Genesis from the Bible. As they orbited the moon, one of the astronauts, William Anders, captured the photograph: *Earthrise*.

And just like that, *Earthrise* became the first scripture of the planetary technotheocracy—an image of such symbolic power that it catapulted society into another liminal space. Whether or not people realized it at the time, there was a clear before and after that first glimpse of Earth from outside.

Its release was timed at a moment of peak social vulnerability—global unrest, war, grief, confusion, longing. Whether by design or coincidence, the image arrived with maximum emotional precision. It bypassed the rational mind and embedded itself directly in the collective subconscious. *Earthrise* wasn't just a photograph. It was a ritual and a symbolic initiation into a new cosmology—one curated not by mystics or sages, but by technicians and screens. It marked the birth of a technocratic mythology, bridging familiar scripture with satellite broadcasting and global awe. The timing was impeccable because the collective was already desperate for escape. When reality becomes too painful, a beautiful illusion can feel like relief.

The image became iconic. It was printed on posters and plastered on walls, eventually becoming the cover of Brand's *Whole Earth Catalog*. That publication sparked a cultural movement, weaving the social vision of the 1960s counterculture with the emerging science of cybernetics.[64,65]

Cybernetics is the science of self-regulating systems, governed by feedback. It quietly became the invisible architecture of the Digital Age. Over the next few decades, it shaped everything from computing to psychology to mechanisms of social control.

Brand began connecting the bohemian communities of San Francisco with the rising tech scene in Silicon Valley. This formed a cultural bridge between psychedelia and programming—a channel through which visionaries and engineers began to dream of planetary transformation through code.

But somewhere along the way a pivot occurred.

What began as a movement for awakening gradually aligned with agendas of control. The dream of personal freedom through technology became a trap. Humans became passive consumers—data points in a growing global grid. Decisions were gradually outsourced to algorithms. Personal data and intimate choices became metrics to analyze.

The human longing to see our planet from above transformed into the surveillance satellite infrastructure encircling the Earth today.

Even the environmental awakening, once inspired by the *Earthrise* image, was hijacked. What began as genuine ecological concern mutated into the climate industrial complex that we see nowadays—a narrative distortion driven by corporate greenwashing, carbon credit capitalism, and technocratic interventions. Global organizations like the World Economic Forum, formed in 1971, positioned themselves as planetary stewards, while quietly centralizing control.

The dream of planetary unification, and the *Earthrise* image—a visual form of art—got co-opted by empire. Or perhaps it was socially engineered from the beginning to do exactly that.

And here's where things get weird. The Central Intelligence Agency (CIA) was formed in 1947, the same year the Department of War was dissolved, and eventually re-branded as the Department of Defense a couple years later. This was a psychological softening of the meaning of war to the implication of defense, as the U.S. expanded military operations.

Allegedly, CIA created Operation Mockingbird in the early years of the Cold War as a covert propaganda program used to influence students and journalists to believe, falsify or embellish stories in order to curate the perception of reality, domestically and abroad. This program allegedly involved the use of bribery and blackmail, among other covert operations. It's also rumored that the agency planted ideas in production studios of Hollywood to spread propaganda via entertainment.

The debate about whether Operation Mockingbird ever existed is still ongoing. Yet nowadays, former CIA officials *openly* appear on mainstream news channels—like CNN—as commentators, sharing their opinions and guiding public discourse.

MKUltra, CIA's top-secret mind control program involving human experimentation took place between 1953 and 1973, at dozens of institutions in the U.S. and Canada including hospitals, prisons, and prestigious universities. Military personnel were also among the subjects of experiments.

The MKUltra program had the aim of developing mind-controlling drugs for the potential use for psychological torture, brainwashing and behavior modification during the Cold War. Many of those experiments violated the Nuremberg Code of informed consent. Some of the subjects were unaware they were dosed with psychedelic substances like lysergic acid diethylamide (LSD). These appear to be a continuation of the Nazi experiments on prisoners in concentration camps. The official end of the MKUltra program was in 1973, one year after the last Apollo moon mission.

The manned moon missions were conducted by the U.S., where 1600 scientists were imported from Nazi Germany in Operation Paperclip after World War II, to gain advantage over the Soviet Union during the Cold War. The aim was to dominate wartime technology. The Nazi scientists in America were primarily working in fields like rocketry and aviation. They were already trained to conform to, and perform under the conditions of, propaganda and lies. They were also already trained to normalize the unethical experimentation on human subjects. Some of the Nazi scientists were hired by NASA and other government agencies. Instead of being held accountable for their war crimes, they were given important jobs. That could be strong leverage to control a person's opinions and actions.

The Smithsonian magazine writes, "While many of the men who were brought to the U.S. under the program were undoubtedly instrumental in scientific advancements like the Apollo program, they were also supportive and responsible for some of the horrors experienced by victims of the Holocaust."[66]

Perhaps all of that is a string of extraordinary coincidences and it was exactly as we were told. Maybe America did send manned missions to the moon in the late 1960s and early 1970s. That's possible. But it's curious that, despite over five decades of exponential technological advancement, it hasn't happened again. The Official Story may be true. But when I consider the psychological landscape of those times—the Cold War tension, the national grief from JFK's and MLK's assassinations, the Vietnam War, the mind control studies, the Nazi scientists working with NASA and other government organizations, the rise of advertising and television as a narrative-guiding force—and how easily perception can be engineered under pressure, I find it more difficult to accept that version without question.

Still, for me, the moon landing itself wasn't the most impactful, long-term inflection point. It was Apollo 8 and the *Earthrise* image. Whether real or manufactured, it revealed something crucial: That art, especially when deployed with precision and timing, has the power to pivot human history. And in the late 1960s, it did.

Then came the depression and psychic shadow of the 1970s culture. Technology advancements and the first computers were the beginning of what would eventually become the Internet and Digital Age. In retrospect, it's becoming clear how these advents made our world appear to be more connected, yet individuals became increasingly more isolated over the following decades.

Now, in our time, we are once again in the peak charge of a planetary turning point. But this time the tools are far more potent and sophisticated. Artificial intelligence. Digital currencies. Biometric surveillance. Climate panic and weather modification. Algorithms that censor information and curate perception. Continuous neurological entrainment with our devices. Social media accelerating psychological manipulation at scale.[67]

A global freedom movement is awakening in response—rightfully sensing the danger. But it too risks being corralled into engineered resistance, just as the counterculture of the 1960s was ultimately absorbed and redirected by the same system it opposed.

AI is increasingly blurring the boundary between what's real and what's manufactured. The rising burden of unresolved trauma makes us more suggestible—primed for influence. If we want to interrupt these ancestral repetition loops, we need to cultivate discernment now more than ever. That means integrating what has gone unprocessed—personally and collectively.

Our *Earthrise* moment is likely approaching—another awe-inducing image or event promising planetary unification. But this time, the fantasy will be much more alluring because the pain of our present is so hard to face.

We can choose differently. We can break the spell of mind control, but not with rebellion. Not through counter-ideologies that inevitably get co-opted to serve the control of the rulership. We need a new way of being human. What's being asked of us now is not resistance. It's restoration. We are being invited to restore the whole self—undivided, unprogrammed, integrated and sovereign.

We are hearing the term Golden Age again recently in America and this ought to perk up our spidey senses. For whom will it be *golden*? We would be wise to be cautious about the fantasies that will likely be sold to us in order to usher us into new forms of social engineering. The social engineers will pluck the strings of fear and play the chords of awe in order to captivate us into the trance. The rush for wartime technology last century opened the door to some very inhumane experiments on people and decades of brainwashing that led our species further into the state of captivity.

In the 2020s and beyond, the wartime rush will entail the use of technology and AI. Ideally, we would develop the technology at a slower pace to allow for responsible and cautious implementation and adoption. However, every major power around the world wants to win the AI race. That urgency is going to lead to recklessness, as it did during the space race of the Cold War when ethics were disregarded and Nazi scientists were imported to win that battle. Yet this time, the stakes are much higher and the risks more unpredictable as the technology is advancing at an exponential rate, and so is the compounding interest burden of our ancestral trauma.

The modern realm of technology also provides another level of possibility for covert experimentation, mind control and plausible deniability. Much of it is invisible—such as the use of radio wave, microwave and millimeter-wave frequencies, which our devices are already using. Every time a new band of frequencies is bombarded into the air, we are participating in an experiment, without safety studies or informed consent. The human brain entrains with frequencies, and this can have vast implications on our health, wellness, sovereignty, behavior and the perception of reality.

Time appears to be moving differently in our era, perhaps less linear and more quantum with the advent of more advanced technologies that are reprogramming our nervous systems. Our ancestors adapted slowly to the advancements in technology of their time. It was nothing like the Digital Age that we are living in now.

Humans are creating technology in the image of our biology. The binary code used by computers is very similar to how our nervous system functions. We have become increasingly more dependent on technology, to the point where most of us are now co-regulating more with our devices than with other humans. While humans are programming technology, technology is reprogramming us.

Children born nowadays are called *digital natives*. A four-year old kid usually knows more about using your smartphone and tablet than you do. That's because she was born with the upgraded tech package in her nervous system, which she inherited from her parents, who were *trained* to use the devices.

Each new generation's biology is becoming more integrated with the technology and vice versa. While many think that transhumanism is something of a far-fetched future, I would assert that the merging of humans and AI is already under way.

The nervous system is the bridge among the body, mind, and spirit. It's also the bridge between humans and technology. The nervous system plays a key role in trauma, connection and healing. We are currently uploading our unresolved trauma into AI and that is going to be reflected back to us in surprising ways.

It's said that history doesn't repeat itself, but that it does rhyme. Our 2020s story already rhymes with the existentially shattering experiences of the entire twentieth century, all combined into a quantum packet of energy in the here and now, due to the added disruption of rapidly advancing technology and the unexpected events that will bring. We are living on the precipice of *a whole new reality*.

Now what?

It has often been said that creativity is the antidote to destruction. In order to bring about personal and social liberation, we will need to take on the responsibility of confronting the darkness within—in our hidden fears, desires, doubts, confusion, pain, and traumas. That is the only way to begin transforming these into sources of insight, strength, wisdom, growth, and light. This is essential if we want to use technology in responsible and beneficial ways.

Can we evolve in a more positive way this time, emerging from the atrocities and trauma of our experiences without repeating the same old cycles, amplified by our new technology?

Can we find a way to integrate the human psyche and society from a state of fragmentation before it's too late?

Can we use art to transcend the painful reality of separation and suffering to discover deeper truths within the subconscious so that we can create a better, lighter, and more conscious path forward?

One thing is for sure, albeit a paradox—our human experience is fractured, yet interconnected. Whether we are aware of it or not, we are all searching for meaning amidst the chaos, trauma, and shock. Here in the shadow of the threshold that leads to our future, we are navigating the liminal spaces together, yet we are also more isolated than ever.

We have the opportunity to seek new ways of making sense of the world, addressing the individual and societal wounds of war, deception, dis-ease, disasters, loss, trauma, scarcity, inner conflicts, and emotional residue. This means we will need to face, digest, metabolize, and process the pain, transforming it through the discovery and integration of profound insights and wisdom that can be extracted like nutrients from the digestive process.

Creating meaning in a chaotic world

André Breton's concept of "convulsive beauty" is about the startling, paradoxical, and breathtaking beauty that emerges from disruption, contradiction, and surprise. Convulsive beauty doesn't conform to trends and mainstream standards, which would be represented by something like Instagram in our time.

Our 2020s standards of beauty involve injecting neurotoxins into our faces as well as toxic fillers into lines, cheeks, and lips, undergoing traumatic plastic surgeries, and using app filters to fix everything else. One day people will look back in awe at how absurd all this was—how it revealed a culture that was afraid to really see itself, with the perfectly imperfect scars of life and all.

Breathtaking beauty arises from tension, unexpected juxtapositions, and even chaos. We age, and our appearance shows the lines and evidence of being alive. Our shape may hollow, sag, and wrinkle in some unsettling ways. Yet when we look into honest eyes, we can observe the wisdom of the receipts of a life lived with pain, mistakes, failures, insecurities, anger, and traumas as well as joy, success, accomplishments, confidence, grace, strength, love, and resilience.

Natural beauty is *convulsive* in an era of faux beauty trends and absurd distortions. Aging is uncomfortable and, of course, most of us would rather look forever young. Yet perhaps the current beauty trends of our culture are representative of how we are the culmination of generations of people avoiding discomfort and reality. We just happen to have the technology to do something material to (pretend to) avoid it.

The surrealism of the twentieth century provided an unusual premise for processing painful experiences through a lens of absurdity, in order to create new meaning from the trauma. What it lacked was the bridge between trauma and purpose, connecting the subconscious and the conscious—the integration.

As with all forms of art, part of the beauty is how it lands for each individual who observes and experiences it. It helps us to make sense of our own experiences and inner life, which was perhaps out of reach before. This is part of the catharsis of emotional expression through art.

The role of playfulness and absurdity can assist in challenging our rigid thinking that gives us a false sense of safety and certainty. It can also help in thawing out the frozen emotions in the muscular armoring often caused by trauma. When things flow, it's easier to reconnect with a sense of wonder and curiosity. Absurd humor can counterbalance the darkness of the experience of trauma, allowing us to *presence* the pain without being overwhelmed by it.

Chaos can be repurposed into something new and meaningful when it is met with presence, curiosity, compassion, courage, and creativity. Art can be a valuable tool in this transformational process because some things are very difficult to talk about and are perhaps more easily expressed and transmuted through artistic mediums.

When we can't talk about it, the self-healing mechanism is blocked. This happens in individuals, families, and society. While talking alone doesn't heal the trauma, as it only engages the conscious mind, it is an important step in the healing process.

The trauma is stored in the subconscious and body. Yet we have to talk about it before we can *start* healing. When insights emerge from the subconscious, then we can continue exploring them through words, language, and verbal understanding. It's all part of the integration.

So here we are in 2025, and society still isn't able to talk about what has happened since 2020. Art can help us to connect with the painful feelings and disturbing reality that we are facing, by starting the conversation and catalyzing the emotional expression and processing.

From these liminal spaces, we have a choice. We can either give up, falling into despair and rescue fantasies that will lead us straight into the technocratic next-level captivity, *or* we can lean into the discomfort of the existential calling of a lifetime in order to come out the other side stronger and wiser than before. Only one of these options leads to empowerment, liberation, and healing for us and future generations. This is our choice.

PART TWO

THE LIBERATION OF SOULS

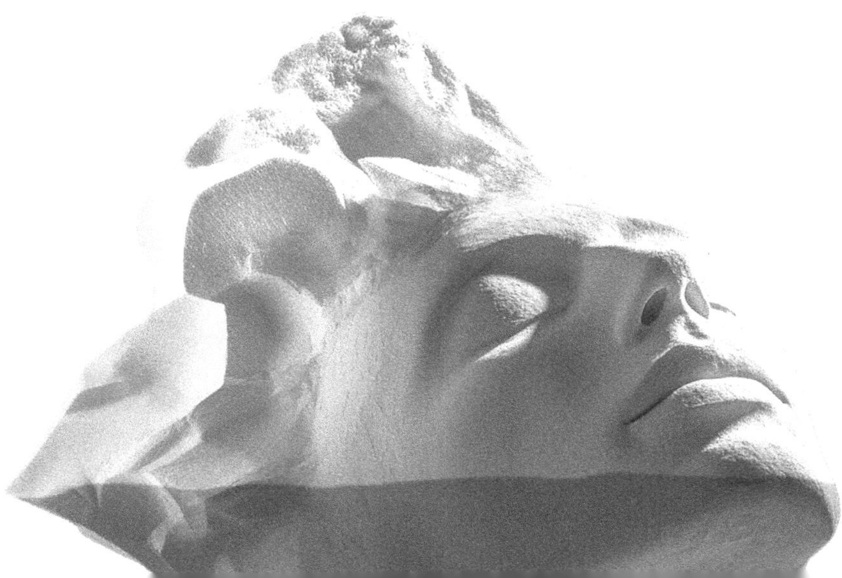

CHAPTER 10

EXPOSING THE DARKNESS

The Great Unveiling

The effects of abuse and tyranny on the human being have holistic implications. In order to understand the individual, we also must take into consideration the physical, emotional, mental, spiritual, social, and technological environment in which the individual exists.

Abuse can only truly be understood and healed through a holistic lens because this is the nature of the human being. The spiritual dimension is one of the most overlooked areas of the human experience when it comes to abuse.

The same applies to tyranny around the globe. We are limiting our understanding of its causes and impact when we simply analyze it through the lens of psychology and rationalism. Evil has spiritual implications.

Psychology is helpful for understanding a bit about the mind and emotions, but that's not the entirety of the human experience, which involves the body–mind–spirit connection. For the same reason, the scientific and medical models of psychology and psychiatry do not have a frame for understanding evil and the effects it has on individuals, couples, family systems, workplaces, and society.

Likewise, modern medicine leaves many questions unanswered. The allopathic medical system is limited by its pixelated perspective of the human being. Most doctors are trained to hyperfocus on a very small sector of the patient's reality, so they miss the big picture.

A holistic lens is necessary to see how it's all connected from the micro level to the macro level. We are each part of that. Transcending the darkness at the individual and collective levels includes addressing the effects of evil and the spiritual realm on the human experience.

It's challenging to expose evil because its nature is deceptive. It takes time for evil to fully reveal itself. We are being permitted to watch this ancient story unfold, in real time, on the global stage and in our personal lives. We are watching evil's mask crack under the pressure of the truth being exposed, yet we still have not seen the full reveal because evil has not reached its culmination. Just like in covert abusive relationships, most people cannot see the evil until it comes into full expression, unveiling itself.

The micro to macro levels of spiritual warfare

Narcissistic abuse is spiritual warfare. This is why the patterns are so similar around the world, regardless of country, culture, race, gender, age, or socioeconomic status. And that's why it can't truly be understood within the limitations of psychology or medicine.

The dark force is not limited by human language and knowledge. It speaks directly to hearts and souls. It knows our deepest fears and insecurities, then uses these against us as they are mirrored through our life experiences.

Those serving the dark forces from the top to the bottom of society don't just want money and power. They are after soul essence. They feed on the stolen life force energy of others because they are disconnected from the divine source of All That Is. Yet something else is feeding off of *them*. Even the perpetrators are enslaved in captivity, though they are usually unwilling to admit it.

Spiritual war is the battle between good and evil. It seems very personal when abuse and demonic oppression is happening. It is highly personalized to the deepest pain, insecurities, and weakness of the individual, family, or society. Yet on another dimension of existence, it's less about the particular people involved and more about the impersonal forces of evil behind the warfare.

A verse from the Bible has been appearing repetitively on my radar since 2020:

> Put on the full armor of God, so that you can make your stand against the devil's schemes. For our struggle is not against flesh and blood, but against the rulers, against the authorities, against the powers of this world's darkness, and against the spiritual forces of evil in the heavenly realms.
>
> Ephesians 6:11–12[68]

The force of darkness is often cloaked in pretty words and behind smokescreens, gaslighting one's true perception. It ensnares people to do its bidding by making them think it's going to alleviate their fears and insecurities. It may do so temporarily, giving a false perception of power, yet it always comes with a cost. Evil flatters and dangles false promises of personal safety and security in exchange for compliance, self-sacrifice, and obedience.

These deceptive promises are positioned as a relief from the intense fear bombardment and perceived inability to escape the soul's state of captivity. It's no wonder so many people are confused and misled while trying to escape their pain and fear. We are living in times of the Great Deception. As Isaiah 5:20 says: "Woe to those who call evil good, and good evil; Who put darkness for light, and light for darkness; Who put bitter for sweet, and sweet for bitter!"[69]

Evil is marketed as virtue, *for your own good* and *for the greater good.* It's been so well disguised in plausible deniability that it's almost believable. And who can dare argue against wanting the good for all?

It's set up to frame *you* as the evil one for questioning it or refusing to comply with the anti-life measures. This force has been dominating humanity for millennia, keeping human souls in generational captivity.

We are now also living in times of exposure and unveiling, as a great awakening is beginning to gather momentum. People, governments, institutions, corporations, and narratives are being revealed for what they really are. Nowadays evil is openly dancing in the streets in plain daylight. More people are waking up as each event unfolds, though not all can see it yet.

With every step the perpetrators take toward their agendas, they are risking overstepping and awakening the masses. More people have been opening their eyes since 2020. The same pattern happens in abusive interpersonal relationships.

However, the force of evil hasn't fully revealed its nature yet. Eventually, more people will see it, as the truth continues to seep through the cracks and things get increasingly more uncomfortable. Of course, there will always be people who refuse to see it, even when it's undeniably visible in front of their faces. With compassion, it's easy to understand why it's so challenging to accept the existence of evil, and why denial seems like a comfortable shelter from reality. However, when we refuse to acknowledge that evil exists in our world, that is a huge liability for falling prey to it—and even enabling it.

The spiritual war isn't new, nor is narcissistic abuse on the interpersonal or societal level. This has probably been happening for all of human history. Perhaps it only seems to be exponentially intensifying as we are reaching a critical evolutionary point in human history.

Many of us were comfortably numb and didn't have any idea what was happening on a micro or macro level until recent years. Topics like narcissistic abuse became more commonly known and a lot of people started joining the online conversation, sharing their life experiences. More people are starting to realize there is a spiritual component to abuse.

Some of us became willing to start looking at these unpleasant phenomena in our personal lives *and* society. It takes bravery to face the ugly truth. It's a lot easier, albeit unhealthy, to live in denial.

It's understandable that some would rather believe evil doesn't exist. Despite the adage of *ignorance is bliss*, not believing in something doesn't make us immune to it—it just makes us blind to what's really happening, and therefore easy targets.

Ignorance usually results in unintended, unfavorable consequences brought about by poor decisions or lack of courageous action when it's most needed. We've all been there at moments, and we can see this currently happening at a collective level in the world.

If a person has not been touched by evil in her personal life (or simply hasn't realized it yet), it's hard to understand that such a thing could exist. Many people still live in a childlike fantasy where all humans are good.

Perhaps we've all had moments of blind innocence in which we believed that all people are inherently good and we just need to be kind to everyone—*love and light, y'all.* This kind of spiritual bypassing can lead people to turn away from the ugly truth and connect with dangerous entities, even doing their bidding.

In spiritual communities we often hear things like, "There's no such thing as good and evil; it's all One." From the perspective of unity consciousness, that's true. Yet it's nuanced. We are also having a human experience on this plane of existence where duality does exist. We would be wise not to ignore or dismiss the full scope of our human experience and the parameters of this world in which we live.

We are witnessing the slow unveiling of evil, layer by layer, and the effects it's having on all of us. That means we are also being forced to turn our gaze *inward*, facing ourselves and our choices with greater honesty and humility.

We are all implicated

Covert abuse becomes overt over time. As it takes on an increasingly more drastic form, it's an opportunity for people to wake up. Many more will be able to identify the darkness in this world, in communities, in families, and in interpersonal relationships as things intensify in our world and in our personal lives.

This awareness also brings the implication that we examine the darkness within ourselves, which is part of our shadow work and spiritual growth. If not, we will unknowingly allow the dark forces to hijack our shadow. Then we can be used as drones to do evil to ourselves and others.

It may be hard to understand how anyone is still sleeping through all the noise, but it's also important to know that some people aren't going to wake up, and that's okay. It's not your job to wake people out of their slumber. It's also not your job to blame, shame, or judge them. This level of compassion is a growing edge for many of us, including myself. It's possible to have compassion *and* boundaries. People will either wake up or not, when and if they're ready, according to their soul contracts. Trying to force their awakening blurs the line of consent.

There is nothing you can say to wake a person from those illusions. You can plant seeds, yet it's only life experience that might one day hit them on the head like a proverbial frying pan, and then they won't be able to unsee it. While unpleasant, those moments are full of divine grace.

Your personal responsibility is to expand your awareness, manage your boundaries, empower yourself through your choices, and liberate yourself from the inner constrictions of the darkness so you can continue to integrate and evolve as a soul, being a lighthouse for others who are still lost in the storm at sea.

Liberating yourself and shining your light of authenticity is the greatest gift you can offer others. The light illuminates the darkness, allowing evil to be seen when it exposes itself. That's not the same as trying to convince or force people to look at it. Do you see the difference? One is an act of service and love. The other is an act of force—a battle of egos, a coping mechanism and distraction from doing the inner work—and *that* is a losing battle.

While the awakening process is ugly and messy at times, it leads to new awareness, which is the initial step to change. First comes the external awareness that evil exists out there. Then comes the more challenging part—the inner awareness of our own participation in the dynamic and the dark shadows within the self. That is the only part we have any control over.

Your power is in your choices. One of the greatest choices you can make in life is to commit to doing the inner work of transmuting the darkness into light.

The dark forces are exposed by the light.

We are living in a time of unveiling. We don't need to fight the darkness. In fact, the more we fight and struggle to control what's trying to control us, the deeper we sink into the quicksand of spiritual despair and existential exhaustion, and the more people will get tricked into turning on one another instead of seeing what's really happening.

Fighting the forces of darkness only makes them stronger. Never argue with demons. It's like food for them, just like what we call *narcissistic supply* in interpersonal relationships. Don't feed the beast. Evil is counting on us falling into this trap. It uses emotional bait to lure us in.

We have the opportunity to triumph by standing courageously in the light of the truth and withdrawing our participation from the lies. The spiritual war out there is a mirror of the *internal* struggle to stand for what is good and to turn away from what is evil.

Our individual choices become our collective, societal circumstances. We have all been participating in some degree of self-deception since long before 2020, and this is why we are living in a world where deception is able to reign, masked as truth.

We've been conditioned to believe that we have no inherent value apart from physical and material symbols of accomplishment, status or beauty, none of which are eternal. We are tricked into devaluing ourselves in the pursuit of false power.

In society, and especially online, we try to prove our value and compete for status, which soothes the ego while we are lured, distracted, and tricked into surrendering more personal dignity as our human rights are covertly controlled or overtly stripped away.

Social media and advertising are full of messages implying unworthiness in order to drive consumer perception and behavior. The algorithm studies your online behavior, mapping your distorted desires and insecurities, then feeds it all back to you. That's why it's called a *feed* when you open up social media platforms. The universe works in a similar way. It also has an algorithm that feeds back to you what you assume to be true through the Law of Assumption.

The dark force tricks us into being pawns for the spiritual war by triggering our wounds, those places inside of us where we feel worthless and powerless. We can easily get caught up in competing or following what everyone else is doing in order to receive social validation and quell these unpleasant feelings of unworthiness.

But everything external is only a temporary reprieve from internal insecurities. It's a futile and endless attempt to fill the inner sense of emptiness. This is how the dark force gets us to entrap ourselves, forgetting that we are free, sovereign beings with inherent worth.

You're unworthy is evil's favorite smear campaign. You probably hear some version of that in intrusive thoughts. Yet this is a lie because worthiness is your divine birthright.

Fear is evil's most powerful tool. The dark force uses fear and doubt to confuse you about who you are and what is true. The essence of that message is to make you believe that you're unworthy so that you can be manipulated. In a state of shame and worthlessness caused by abuse, it is all too easy to lose faith in yourself, in the Creator of All That Is, and in life.

When all faith is lost and spiritual bankruptcy sets in, things become dire. The greatest pain is when we feel disconnected from God. You are so worthy of the Creator's love and you are part of All That Is.

The light is truth, awareness, information, love

The darkness is the absence, corruption, perversion, and distortion of all the above.

A spirit of deception has long ago infected the world, drawing people into its trance—perpetuating the lies, hiding the truth or turning us away from it, spreading misinformation, confusion, and hatred—all the while accusing others of doing those very things.

This is called projection, and it's often what abusers and their enablers do. Any of us can project when we don't want to see the shadow within because it's easier to blame someone else when we are suppressing the pain.

The victim consciousness is an infection of darkness, like a demonic oppression. It tricks us into believing we are powerless. Evil can only maintain its dominance when we believe that it's more powerful than the light of our consciousness. Many of us are the generational curse-breakers, rising above this old story on behalf of our families and ancestral lineage.

The darkness confuses the minds and hearts of the people. Any of us can be brainwashed by spiritual warfare when we are not standing in our integrity and inner power. We've all been there at some point.

The longer the confusion goes on, the more those seeds of doubt will sprout and propagate like unattended weeds in a garden. Perception becomes further distorted until the point when a person can lose complete touch with reality, becoming fully subscribed to the lies, while believing they are truths. By that point, it will require an ego death to face the truth. And that requires strength of character.

While the spiritual war is not new, never has there been a more direct assault upon the soul of humanity, than now in the post-2020 world, to reduce the population and usher us into the next level of captivity, through technology.

If you're reading this book, you're likely already aware of that to some degree. But if you've been lacking a community of kindred spirits, you might be doubting yourself or your perspective of reality. That can cause you to dim your light in order to feel safe.

I want to encourage you to shine your light brightly and ignore those who tell you to turn it down for their comfort. Shine, baby, shine! You are a spark of the Divine. Start acting like it and you'll be able to laugh at the absurdity of the lies.

It's no coincidence that abusers in interpersonal relationships use these same tactics of whittling down the target's self-worth until she is collapsed, numb, frozen, shutdown, debilitated, and disconnected from self, loved ones, and God, while becoming increasingly more dependent on the abuser for survival.

The abuse doesn't work if we know we are worthy. Your self-worth is your greatest immunity to abuse, use, deception, and manipulation. We will explore that more in Chapter 14.

The world is going down a very tumultuous path that perhaps one day will be described as the greatest deception in human history with catastrophic generational consequences.

Or perhaps we will choose a different path leading toward regeneration, making this a story of redemption and deliverance.

Either way, in retrospect, the 2020s will certainly be noted as another historical turning point, like great wars and cataclysms in the past—a death-and-rebirth cycle, a clear before and after.

Which way do we go from here?

That's the big question and it depends on the sum of our individual choices and actions.

Much like our challenging personal transformation cycles when we are put through the fire of spiritual purification in order to find greater purpose and meaning, eventually, something good will come of this, too. In retrospect, more people will realize this was all happening *for* us, not to us.

But first it will get uglier.

Over the years I've noticed that only a small percentage of victims of narcissistic abuse end up doing the challenging inner work required for the self-healing process. Most people never get past the self-honesty part in order to shift into the commitment of owning personal responsibility over their choices and life.

First, we must admit what we are doing and how we are participating in our own captivity in order to go through the inner reckoning process toward liberation.

It can feel very relieving at first to discover information about the abusers and manipulators in your life and on the global stage. Yet that can become a trap if we stay stuck in the early stage of healing, learning all about what the other person (or people) did.

While it's challenging to accept the existence of evil in the world, that's the easier part. Many people get stuck in that phase of awakening, focusing on the external. They are unable, or unwilling, to cross the threshold of commitment to self-responsibility in order to step into empowerment and transform their lives. This shift requires looking within and shining a light on the inner darkness so that we can integrate our shadow instead of running from it or projecting it outward.

Likewise, we will probably also see a small percentage of society thriving through this transformational cycle of the 2020s. It will require doing the inner shadow work, not just having the external awareness of evil in the world as well as the injustice and harm that was done *to* humanity. This perspective will keep us in the victim consciousness.

Currently, the dark forces acting through those on the world stage are desperately trying to maintain control over the minds and hearts of the people. They're hurried and desperate because they know they're losing their grip, and that their era of ruling is ending. The energetic shifts in our cosmos are causing more of us to awaken.

The *beings without conscience inhabited by evil entities playing good*, and the invisible force of darkness that they serve, will continue to use more intimidation and fear tactics because they are terrified that we are waking up and turning away from the lies, illusions, and deception.

They are not afraid of being exposed. As Carlos Castaneda asserted, *petty tyrants* are most afraid of being insignificant. And we have been giving them entirely too much significance.

They are panicked that a growing number of us are unsubscribing from the narrative, withdrawing our participation, and not reacting as they expected. They feel entitled to get away with it, and their grandiosity has them convinced that they will. So, they're hurried now to push their agenda forward. Their pride will eventually be their downfall.

Likewise, hubris is our greatest challenge to breaking free from the state of captivity in which most of humanity has lived for so long. As entrepreneur and podcaster Taylor Welch says, the kryptonite for humans is pride.

It's often said that it's darkest before the dawn. Perhaps this intense pressure in our world and personal lives now is the motivation we needed to empower ourselves and transmute our wounds into light.

Evolutionary pressure is building

We are seeing things escalate now. A covert abuser meticulously attacks every pillar of the target's life: family, friendships, work performance, ability to earn income, physical and mental health, spiritual connection, the freedom of movement, and expression.

Yet for the total destruction to be effective, abusers must disconnect the targets from their support system and isolate them from outside perspectives. That's why the first parameter of the state of captivity is isolation from outside perspectives—a key part of the ongoing trauma that's taking place now in society.

This cycle will continue to escalate into more open assault on human rights, the human spirit, our individual sovereignty, and our God-given right to exist in this world.

Many clients I've worked with who grew up in families with narcissistic abuse have a core wound and belief that says "I don't have the right to exist." This is what tyrants want us to believe, because when we believe that, it becomes our reality and we see everything through that lens.

The evil forces will keep destroying the fabric of society, pillar by pillar, just as a psychopath destroys the victim's life in an interpersonal relationship. The sooner we turn away from evil in our own lives, the better. The longer it goes on, the more difficult it is to get out.

All of this leaves many of us wondering, why does our Creator allow such evil to exist?

What if it's all a calling back to God?

Perhaps the existence of evil is like a spiritual alarm clock calling us to turn away from the toxic distractions, lies, deceptions, illusions, and emptiness, instead turning toward what is good and real. Maybe it's waking us up so we can see our true nature as human beings, free from the distortions and corruption of this world.

What if it's all evolutionary pressure calling us toward the liberation of the human soul?

This is the greatest opportunity that the dark forces offer. No one can *take away* your power, but you can be tricked into *giving* it away. It can be challenging to accept that personal responsibility, especially if you've been disempowered for most of your life, as I was. We've been conditioned through ancestral programming and ongoing social conditioning to give our power away to feel safe, to fit in, to be accepted.

We've been tricked into fighting what we don't want and focusing our energy on those very things, which only feeds and strengthens those forces. That can be a challenging reality to accept, but it's a doorway to greater empowerment when you realize that this is a choice. It's your choice. And that's where you'll find your power.

After decades of abusive relationships, this is what I've come to understand as the higher purpose of encounters with evil. It all forced me to wake up to my own dysfunctional habits and patterns—to see my own shadow and how I was enabling the dark forces in my life. It wasn't my fault that I was programmed that way due to childhood and ancestral trauma from my lineage. But it is my responsibility what I'm doing about it now. Observing these same abuse patterns in the world, I feel like this is a calling for humanity, too.

We can choose to accept the invitation of evil or not. This means we can choose to enable the darkness and feed it or not. We can choose to allow it to destroy us. Or we can see how it's a higher calling to evolve.

The spiritual war isn't just out in the world. It's taking place inside the hearts and minds of each of us. What we see in the external world is a reflection of the collective sum of our inner worlds.

We ought to learn to discern the evil surrounding us and also that possibility which exists within the choices given to each of us at any moment. This isn't about shaming ourselves. It isn't happening because we are bad or unworthy. It isn't a punishment, judgment or blame. It's happening *for* us to recognize the opportunity to grow and evolve.

Our individual choices are creating the kind of world we are living in. There is no fixing the world or saving the country. The external focus is a bypassing and avoidance of what we can control. The transformational work starts inside each of us and ripples outward.

The spiritual virus

Before the radical changes in the world started in 2020, I used to think the pandemic was narcissism and psychopathy, as if these phenomena were the contagious illness in society. Now I realize that the perpetrators of darkness are infected with something like a spiritual virus and the dis-ease they cause is disconnection. They use many trauma-based tactics to isolate people, to divide and conquer the masses, to create a fragmentation in society and a separation of the individual from self, others and the Creator of All That Is.

After the first several years of this global shift taking place, I'm realizing that the plandemic was more about the disconnection caused by abuse and isolation, and the spiritual force of darkness that drives it.

There are many influences contributing to the contagion of disconnection. For example, the news, entertainment, social media, algorithms, unresolved and ongoing trauma, and our increasing dependence on technological devices and the effects of these on the human nervous system. At the core, trauma creates fear, scarcity, and separation.

The perpetrators use all the above as tools to isolate individuals, while giving us the illusion of being connected. We are coerced into identifying with a group for safety, and from there it's easy to divide and conquer society.

There's a growing sense of disconnection happening in society and within individuals. The isolation isn't just physical. It also plagues the human mind and soul. The more invisible dimensions of loneliness are perhaps the most devastating.

If you've experienced loneliness in a relationship, family, workplace, social group, or even when living in a big city surrounded by millions of people, you can probably relate to how devastating that feels. *People, people everywhere and not a connection in sight.*

It's possible, and even a common experience, to be surrounded by people without feeling a safe, real, and deep connection. In those cases, it can feel lonelier with people than when alone.

While it can be helpful, relieving, and validating to connect with people online, our interactions through social media and other aspects of digital life are not the same as real-life human connection. The addiction to external validation via social media is the new alcoholism normalized as culture.

Remember this in the coming years when the manipulators try to sell us the metaverse and virtual reality as a replacement for, or augmentation of, real human connection. They will use words like "socialization" and "more connected" to make it sound nice, but these are illusions.

As ridiculous as it sounds, it's going to appear very attractive to escape real life and enter the virtual reality of fantasy. If you think that many people are disconnected from reality now, just wait until this becomes a commonly acceptable form of escape! It will lead to more captivity.

Maybe you can relate to feeling like you're living in an entirely different reality than others. The wild thing is that we all believe our reality is real. Perception is reality.

As more truth comes out and shatters the illusions we've held for generations, we are quickly being re-directed into the next narrative of distorted reality where all is forgotten in a spectacular display of surrealism.

The metaverse combined with the Internet of Bodies (IoB)[70] is going to bring a whole other level of insanity and delusional psychosis as people voluntarily plug themselves into the matrix and, over time, lose touch with real life, human connection, their inherent worthiness and individual sovereignty. It will be disguised as "improving human wellness."

Earlier in this book we explored the devastating disconnection from self, others, and God caused by the fear programming and traumatic experiences. As countries, communities, and families are becoming more splintered, individuals are becoming more isolated.

What is the increasing sense of disconnection doing to the soul of humanity?

What will be the implications for future generations if we don't change trajectories?

We've all become more reliant on digital means of communication for work and personal life. The COVID narrative has ushered us into a new way of digital life. It's amazing that we can communicate with each other around the world thanks to technology. Yet we are becoming accustomed to less in-person interaction. This is part of the social engineering process leading us into a more distanced and virtual world. The longer we are disconnected, the more challenging it is to reconnect.

I'm unsure at what point the disconnection can alter our species permanently, because this has never been done before. I'll admit it's creepy that the youngest generation, the one that follows Gen Z, was named Generation Alpha. The beginning of what? A new human prototype that is merging with technology?

The real plandemic is the disconnection

Years from now, we will look back at the early 2020s and realize that it wasn't the virus that inflicted the highest toll on human life. That was a deception. It was the weaponization of fear and its fallout on the physical, psychological, spiritual, technological, behavioral, and social life of the human being.

The disconnection started, mostly invisibly, decades before the 2020s. Social isolation has been increasing slowly over time with the accumulation of unresolved trauma, the adoption of technology, and the ways humans have adapted to it.

Our brains and bodies are changing through our exposure to technology, which is having implications for other areas of human life. One of the areas that appears to be most affected is social bonding.

In recent years, public "health" policies have been greatly exacerbating the social isolation and causing many more problems than they're solving. However, the truth is now being revealed.

Researchers at Johns Hopkins University—the same institution that collected and reported data on COVID case counts, death counts, and jab doses administered until 2023—concluded that lockdowns had no noticeable effect on reducing COVID-related deaths and instead had a devastating effect on economies and created many social ills.

Health News Florida brought this study to light:

> "We find no evidence that lockdowns, school closures, border closures, and limiting gatherings have had a noticeable effect on COVID-19 mortality," researchers wrote in the report…
>
> The study concluded that lockdowns "are ill-founded and should be rejected as a pandemic policy instrument."
>
> "They have contributed to reducing economic activity, raising unemployment, reducing schooling, causing political unrest, contributing to domestic violence, and undermining liberal democracy," the report said.[71]

The perpetrators didn't accept accountability or express remorse for what they did, even though this truth is already being revealed along with the many harms caused by the injections. Instead, they evaded the reckoning, acted like nothing happened, and quickly pivoted to the next crisis—war.

Due to the ongoing propaganda, fear of the other is replacing a sense of human connection. It was hard to pinpoint exactly what was going on in society before all this ramped up some years ago. But there was definitely something happening before anyone ever heard the word COVID.

I could sense it as early as 2010 or so when I observed people at social gatherings, or with their family and friends in restaurants, bars and cafes, or even couples on dates. Looking around, most people were doing something on their phone, creating disconnection and absence instead of connection and presence.

There was a palpable sense of disconnection in the interactions, even among the laughs and loud voices. *Something was missing.*

Of course, there have always been some deeper human connections no matter what is going on in the world. I experience this with my closest friends, and I've observed these sorts of connections in public, albeit very rarely.

Maybe you have some true connections in your life, too. These are the relationships of authentic substance. There is a reciprocal presence. Even if you disagree, you can speak about real things, even controversial topics, without feeling like you have to hide your authenticity, dim your light, or walk on eggshells to avoid the landmines of guardedness, defensiveness, judgment, image management, and fakery.

In real connections, you can feel a deeper sense of shared experience, presence, and emotional and spiritual intimacy rather than just superficial small talk or hiding behind devices. These are the connections that let the light in and amplify it.

During recent years, we've been invited to look within and see what really matters. This has been one of the greatest gifts of these intense times. It's an invitation to clarify our personal core values so we can align our internal holistic connection of body–mind–spirit, and restore our authentic connection with God and other people. Yet the dis-ease of disconnection must be addressed internally first, in order to change the way we connect with others.

The internal spiritual alignment and coherence makes it much easier to find the right relationships and allies in order to move through these challenging times together and rebuild with afterward. We have been drifting apart slowly, yet increasingly, for decades. The plandemic of disconnection in our world is a calling for true connection.

Connection is the antidote to disconnection

When we connect wholeheartedly with self, others, and the Creator of All That Is, something miraculous happens. These experiences metaphysically connect us with a spiritual force much bigger than us as individuals.

When we experience the wholeness of authentic and deep connection, something magical happens, yet this is a natural part of who we are as holistic beings. We've mostly forgotten because it isn't trending in pop culture, it's often not spoken of in families, and we surely don't see it in the news.

Some of us have traveled to remote places on this planet to connect with teachers and mystics who opened us to such experiences. Initially, it can be helpful to leave the comforts and familiarity of home and routine to leap into the possibility of new experiences in which we can catch glimpses of the ineffable. A deep connection with All That Is feels like remembering who we really are.

Have you ever had that kind of indescribable depth of connection when you felt like you were inseparably part of everything, realizing that it's all singing, dancing, and breathing together—and you are part of it all?

The desire for communion with All That Is comes from the human spirit. The need for connection with others of our species is built into our nervous system as mammals. It reads cues of safety, then promotes homeostasis and self-healing through the act of co-regulation—a reciprocal witnessing of each other via eye contact, facial expressions, and sometimes physical touch. Of course it's also important to choose these connections wisely, lest we expose ourselves to more abuse and harm.

Abusers and tyrants isolate us and make us afraid of one another. They restrain personal liberties and human rights much more easily when we are divided and conquered. That's not the path to safety, even though they tell us *they just want to protect us.*

Social distancing does not create a sense of safety in the human nervous system, even though they tell us *staying apart keeps us together*.

The physiological, psychological, and spiritual consequences of the trauma of disconnection aren't temporary if left untreated. It's already leaving an imprint on us and we ought to be taking this seriously.

Many children nowadays will likely grow up without understanding what happened to them during their formative years. They don't know why it's so hard for them to make friends. Without the wisdom, safety, and protection of adults leading the way, how can these children make up for the developmental interruptions or heal from the devastating sense of disconnection that programmed their brain and nervous system in early life?

Having social connections with others with whom we feel safe, share core values, and can verify reality together is an important part of our recovery process and a valuable inspiration to restore our light. This is also a key component of thriving through the intensity of the time we are living in now.

Social connection was wired into our nervous system so we can have mutual healing experiences through the presence of others. On the one hand, there's the mammalian neurological co-regulation. In addition, there's a powerful sharing of energetic codes that happens as humans when we transmute layers of our darkness into light.

I've experienced this phenomenon more recently with some people I've encountered in work and life. As one person shifts a packet of dark energy into light, those liberated light codes are shared with the other person, which catalyzes an energetic activation. Then later that day or over the next few days or weeks, both people experience new inspiration, clarity, or creativity.

This effect is not the same as merely talking and sharing conscious information. That can inspire new ideas and thoughts. But it's a whole other level of energetic activation and liberation that happens when we share light codes. Yet this is only possible as we heal ourselves. When we are in a disempowered state of victim consciousness, we get triggered instead of activated. We need to be in a state of empowerment to get the activation.

When we are unable to feel connected with others, that sense of disconnection makes us more susceptible to spiritual attack. When distance is created instead of connection, that's an open invitation to the dark forces to come in and fill the void.

When we aren't approaching our connections with sincerity, presence, and conscious intention—and instead with fear, hatred, or walls of defensiveness—that creates ambiguity, absence, resentment and distance, which eventually grows into a great divide, much as we see in society as well.

Confusion is usually the first sign of the darkness invasion. It's subtle at first but then becomes more intense and pervasive. This feeling of confusion grows over time, making a person feel isolated, alone, and misunderstood.

This can even happen between two good people who love each other but are unaware of the dark forces manipulating their ability to communicate and connect. That's usually due to unresolved past trauma that gets triggered without the awareness of what's happening.

People can begin to see one another as the enemy instead of realizing that the darkness is confusing them. They might argue or attack one another instead of realizing where the spiritual attack is coming from and how it's hijacking their shadow.

It's best to clear up any confusion immediately with honest, direct communication before it gets worse. When you communicate to get greater clarity and another person responds with more ambiguity, silence, evasion, defensiveness, stonewalling, or contempt, that's not a good sign. It may mean that clarity and connection isn't possible at that time with that person.

Disconnection is intentionally caused in abusive systems through triangulation and the divide-and-conquer tactic. This game in society is clearer now than ever. The result is the unprecedented polarity we are seeing around the world. The perpetrators reward people for participating in the black-and-white narratives that divide us. Every narrative has two sides, neither of which is the whole truth, in order to keep us arguing and seeing one another as the enemy instead of realizing how we are being manipulated from the top down. We are punished by the perpetrators for gathering in unity and we are smeared by enablers on both sides of the narrative when we recognize and speak about the nuance. There is usually some truth on each side of a narrative, as well as distortion.

The same story is happening all over the world, tailored to the local, cultural, and historical themes of wounding. In some places the division wound is most painful when related to skin color and gender, while in other areas it's more about socioeconomic class, religion, or something else. The dark forces know our greatest vulnerabilities, pain, and insecurities.

People are being driven apart in too many ways for this to be a coincidence. It's all part of social engineering, which follows the patterns of spiritual darkness.

Fighting each other is a trap. This is how we participate in our own disconnection and demise. *Divide and conquer* is a weapon of mass distraction. It's a favorite tool of the dark forces.

Mattias Desmet, professor of psychology at the University of Ghent in Belgium, says that in a totalitarian system, there is only one social bond permitted—that of the state with the individual. I would add that the dark forces use the same tactic at the spiritual level, allowing us only to bond with *the authorities, the powers of this world's darkness, the spiritual forces of evil in the heavenly realms.*

The more the social engineers try to drive us apart, the more important it is to cultivate a healthy connection with our true self, others, and the Creator of All That Is.

When we recognize, restore, and harness the potential of human connection, this becomes a powerful antidote to the lies and other spiritual warfare tactics. When we can connect in healthy ways, we amplify the light that continues to expose the shadow in ourselves and the darkness in our world so we can become more aware and bring in more light to restore wholeness.

CHAPTER 11

THE TRUTH WILL SET US FREE

The Quest for Liberty

How is it that we are living in a world where massive lies can survive so long, and what can we do about it?

I had been thinking about this during the peak of COVID tyranny, when one of my neighbors posted something in a local group that stopped me in my tracks: "Healing takes place when we are truthful with God, with ourselves and with others. Maybe you're trying to pretend that you're fine. You can lie to yourself. But God knows you. He knows where you truly are and he knows how to get you to where you need to be in life."

I realized I was so preoccupied with the lies happening out in the world that I wasn't paying attention to how I was lying to myself. And that was why I was stuck.

Honesty starts within. Being honest and truthful with ourselves and others feels vulnerable. It can be scary even when your expression of truth is well received and respected by others. It's much scarier when people hate you for speaking the truth. The latter is usually what happens when people speak up about abuse dynamics in relationships, family systems, other social groups, and society.

Speaking the truth requires discernment about when, how, and with whom to speak. It also requires courage to be honest, even when it's just an internal conversation you're having with yourself.

Of course it's not safe to be truthful, open, and vulnerable with abusers and manipulators. They'll use that against you. Abuse does serious damage to trust and truthfulness. Inevitably, people leave those situations with a devastating trust wound. You can lose trust in yourself, in others, and even in God because you're left wondering: How could such things happen?

To heal the trust wound, you're going to need a guide who knows the terrain because he's been there and can show you a path to freedom. Otherwise, you're going to stumble around in the dark, suffering unnecessarily like I did. When people share the wisdom of their experience, you can learn from their mistakes and insights without having to go through the same painful process.

The challenge is that the trust wound often becomes personified in untrustworthy people who do more harm and add to the pain. The other big challenge comes from the self-sabotage and self-harm programs that usually kick in *just* when you're starting to heal and make progress. Both of these pitfalls happen when we aren't being honest with ourselves.

You learn to doubt yourself and your perception of reality due to the abuse. You start to believe the lies that are directly taught to you or indirectly inferred through the way people treat you. You can end up internalizing other people's thoughts, feelings, emotions, opinions, and perceptions of reality, as well as their pain and projections.

That can make you feel safer in an unsafe environment, but then it becomes confusing what's yours and what isn't. So, you lie to yourself more every day about why that relationship or situation is okay and what it means about you. You might convince yourself that you're fine, but deep down you know it's not true.

When we are honest about how we feel in a relationship or situation, we will honor the totality of our experience of it. That means we won't unconsciously go into defensive states like people-pleasing, suppressing our thoughts and emotions, rationalizing why the relationship or situation is okay, or shutting down and going along with it while checking out of our body. It also means we won't be going into a fight state where we lash out in pain and anger toward someone else or direct it inward in acts of brutality toward the self.

We are starting to see the long-term impact of the wounding to trust that it's taking place around the world due to the massive amount of lies that are being positioned as truth, as well as the casualties of psychological and spiritual war and abuse.

We are living in a world that, for the most part, is going on with life like nothing happened between 2020 and 2022. *But it did happen.* We are collectively pretending it was fine. *But it was not.* We are lying to ourselves and not honoring our experience of what happened. This is not a path toward healing and integrating the past. It's also not the way to prevent it from happening again.

As the disruptive truth continues to come out layer by layer, there will be a growing epidemic of mental illness as people are being confronted with what they'd rather pretend isn't true. Retreating into mental illness is one way to avoid reality and maintain the state of captivity.

When the ego isn't strong enough to face the embarrassment of being wrong and admitting it without getting crushed under the weight of shame, that can keep people doubling down on their illusions and fantasies. It's easier to go on like nothing happened, but the denial eventually comes with a massive cost.

I spoke with a geriatric doctor in Australia who is paying attention to what happened around the world. She confirmed a suspicion that I've had from observing many stories of narcissistic family systems, including my own. Where there is denial of abuse and trauma for decades, dementia often sets in.

The doctor told me she also observed this phenomenon in her practice among elderly patients who were keeping secrets for many years, such as experiencing domestic abuse or lying for decades to their kids about the identity of their real father.

Since 2021, the geriatric doctor has been observing an alarming increase in what she calls "turbo dementia" among her patients. This may be a symptom of the experimental injections as well as the forced isolation and abuse of elders during those years—yet another tragic consequence of the lies and deception campaign.

Like many of us, this doctor wonders when justice is going to happen for the crimes against humanity. Almost all her medical colleagues are pretending like everything is fine, though an occasional one will admit in private to seeing an alarming increase in cardiovascular disease and other maladies among patients. However, the doctor noticed that these colleagues won't talk about *why* that could be happening, and they won't *publicly* admit that it's happening at all.

One of the obstacles that prevents people from seeing the truth is not wanting to know that such evil exists in the world, and that some of the very people they trust are cut from that cloth.

The mandate of silence

It is said that the truth will set us free. Why is that? Many people experience incredible adversity for speaking the truth.

If you tried to tell the truth in an abusive family, workplace, or other social circle, you probably realized that people don't want to believe you. In fact, they will usually turn on you, saying that you're spreading fear or lies. *You're* the one destroying the family. What they mean is you destroyed the *image* they had of the perfect family, which is part of their own ego and identity. Your questioning of their reality feels like a life threat because facing the truth means the death of the false self.

Taking a stand for the truth is one of the scariest things you'll ever do. People who speak the truth about abuse are not socially rewarded in an abusive system.

Speaking the inconvenient truth causes all the alarm bells to sound in the matrix. When you talk about abuse in a family, workplace, or other social system, people will immediately turn on you, even some you never expected to betray you. These might be the people closest to you and who stood by your side in the past. They'll attack you in order to defend the illusions that they're desperately clinging to. This is because they're terrified that they can't survive without the abuser, the abusive system, or the fantasy that they really want to believe in.

It may come as a shock when that happens, and it can be devastating to lose one's social support. Many people experienced this when they questioned the COVID narrative, chose not to wear masks, or chose not to get vaxxed. The same happens when people have strong ego attachments to politicians, political parties, corporations, religious institutions, sports teams, or celebrities.

Enablers defend abusers because they're dependent on the abuser and the system (such as the family, office, or social group) for their sense of self as well as other resources. They want you to silence yourself so they can keep living in their fantasy world. If you don't voluntarily silence yourself, they will try to silence you with love-bombing, smear campaigns, stonewalling, humiliation, blame-shifting, shaming, and other tactics.

The absence of truth caused by the mandate of silence is an open invitation to the dark forces that thrive in environments of lies, illusions, deception, distortion, fantasy, and confusion. It's fear that keeps us subscribed to the mandate of silence, and it's the courage to speak and name things that starts the healing process.

Nowadays, as a result of decades of social engineering, and even more so since the advent of social media, it's easy to drift into the lies and illusions. We've all developed a propensity toward some form of *disordered love*, as Dante Alighieri referred to pride, envy, lust, greed, wrath, sloth, and gluttony. These distorted desires block our clear perception of what is true and false. It's how we become lost in life. A lost soul is its own worst enemy.

We've been seduced, groomed, conditioned, and programmed to love the lie, to indulge in illusion and to adopt distorted desires that lead us away from freedom and true love. Yet we also have choices and free will.

Most of society is oblivious to the effect of social engineering, smartphones and other devices, media, advertising, and culture because it's so normalized. It's easy to assume that our thoughts, opinions, and worldview are our own. Most of us have no idea how much our perception has been molded and shaped by outside forces. None of us is completely immune to this.

We ought to be paying attention because AI is advancing exponentially now. The blur between what is true and what isn't is becoming more pronounced. Energetic discernment is a vital life skill for recognizing external influences and unsubscribing from what is not ours. It's also key for identifying our own distorted desires and restoring healthier forms of love.

In Dante's *Divine Comedy*, he realizes during his journey toward freedom that a vital part of his growth comes through facing the truth about his distorted desires. Like Dante, most of us have become lost and bruised by cowardice. That's right where I found myself in early 2020. The COVID tyranny was a wakeup call to get my desires in order.

Shifting away from the fear and fantasy

In the media, we see a continual use of fear bombardment, now quickly pivoting from one narrative to another in rapid fire, to keep people overwhelmed, disempowered, shut down, apathetic, and compliant.

Speaking the truth with others who can hold space for that level of truth starts to reduce the fear, which weakens the state of captivity. The fear is the glue of the trauma bond.

Initially you might feel dread when you speak up. Dread is the crushing fear that you're going to get in trouble for telling the truth, even when you're talking with people who understand. This is just a remnant of the mandate of silence and the fear of being exiled, ostracized, or annihilated for telling the truth.

If your experience of speaking the truth is met with invalidation, shaming, guilt-tripping, or other adverse reactions from your family or social circle, you might talk yourself out of what you know to be true because it's too painful to deal with. This is how we can end up gaslighting ourselves due to other people gaslighting us.

When you realize that you can't speak the truth with certain people in your life, it's natural to start to distance yourself from them so you can live in the truth. In some cases, you might realize you need to go completely *no contact* with certain people in order to maintain your sanity, health, and wellbeing. This boundary is up to you, but you should have the least amount of contact possible with abusive people. The only way to maintain your sanity while staying in abusive social systems is to suppress the truth, which will have long-term detrimental holistic health effects.

In many cases, the no-contact boundary also involves the enablers, who will abuse you by proxy due to their loyalty to the abusers. You might have some painful experiences of walking away from people you love because you're unable to live in the truth, love yourself, *and* maintain those relationships.

It's very difficult to make that choice because of the emotional attachment to the person or people, and because the autonomic nervous system is seeking connection to feel safe. However, in the case of abuse, those attempts to connect are unhealthy and unsafe.

The truth helps us to face and resolve inner conflicts so that the healing can take place. Before resolving the cognitive dissonance caused by the intermittent reinforcement that we explored in Chapter 2, you might notice that you go in and out of denial about the truth. You might consciously know that you've been abused for some time before the subconscious denial finally shatters. You'll feel it viscerally when it does.

Inner conflicts create dissonance, which causes an energetic distortion pattern that disturbs your ability to function coherently in life. As soon as the truth is observed and accepted at a visceral level, the dissonance dissolves. The truth becomes an instantaneous relief from the gnawing internal tension and struggle that had been maintaining the conflict.

The visceral acceptance of the truth is what inevitably dissolves the cognitive dissonance. This will happen spontaneously during a moment of moving from breakdown to breakthrough. If you're struggling with this, you can be working in that direction by *relentlessly facing the truth* as often as possible. Call yourself out on the lies you hear in your Inner Dialogue and notice when you're slipping into the fantasy or illusion of what you want to believe in, which keeps you stuck in the cycle.

If we are honest with ourselves, we can see when we are holding on to a fantasy of what could be or the potential of a friendship or a relationship, when that's not the reality. It's not always an immediate insight. In fact, there's usually a delayed reaction to this recognition because the flight into fantasy gets triggered in order to adapt to the freeze state.

Those of us who experienced childhood abuse and neglect are more prone to fleeing into fantasy as a defense mechanism because that's what helped us to feel safe when we were defenseless children in an inescapable situation.

For example, during the sexual abuse by my grandfather when I was very young, I instinctually created a fantasy that he loves me. Surely that helped me to survive and feel safe at the time. However, in adulthood that fantasy was still happening in my relationships. Even though I consciously know the difference between sexual interest and emotional intimacy, I didn't have access to my conscious mind when the trauma program got triggered. When someone would show sexual interest in me, or tell me that he loves me while abusing me, my brain would run the "he loves me" program. That led me to have many painful experiences before I could consciously catch myself and reverse-engineer what happened and change the pattern.

Letting go of a fantasy involves facing the truth and then processing the grief of the loss of what we wanted to believe was true. Yet even in such a painful process, there's a sense of a burden being alleviated by the light of the truth. This bittersweetness feels relieving and liberating. It's also quite unsettling because we were used to the illusions and the truth is something new, like fresh skin formed after a wound heals.

The sword of truth

The more willing we are to face ourselves, the easier it is to be honest with ourselves. If we are consistently honest with ourselves and others, it becomes clearer when we are dealing with people who are lying.

Sometimes people lie to deceive. Other times people lie to avoid an internal confrontation with the truth. Usually, we are lying to ourselves and don't even know it.

When the truth is absent from a relationship, what we find is defensiveness, distance, and disconnection. Whether a person is unaware that she's lying to herself or consciously pretending, the result is very similar.

Where there isn't truth, that's not real love, and intimacy cannot grow there. Defensiveness, distance, and disconnection are not the foundation of a healthy relationship with self, others, society, or God.

When we lie to ourselves, we aren't present. Instead of presence, there is an absence that creates an opening for the dark forces to enter.

When a person isn't present with you, you won't feel safe with her and vice versa. Usually, our relationships are a mirror of how we aren't being honest and present with ourselves, so we can notice where we are stuck.

Telling the truth is love. The truth is the source from where love emerges. Being truthful is how healthy relationships are formed with God, with oneself, and with others.

If a relationship is not based on the truth, it's not love. Without the truth, it inevitably drifts into fantasy, illusion, delusion, distortion, deception, lies, and confusion.

When we experience betrayal from the people who were closest to us, especially in childhood, we usually learn not to be honest with ourselves about those painful experiences. When we can't honor our experience in our family, we will do the same in relationships and other areas of our life. We might prefer to live in a beautiful illusion than see the ugly truth. That's where the unhealed betrayal wound becomes self-betrayal.

We are living in a world where pretense is more common than the truth. Social media has greatly emphasized this trend. It's a challenge to stay honest in a climate of lies, illusions, and fantasies. That's even more true if you were trained by your family to say that you're fine, to pretend you want to do whatever they coerce you to do, so you can stay connected and avoid punishment.

Each of us contributes as part of the whole. If lies are ruling the world with such ease, it's because we have drifted from the truth, individually and collectively, for this to be possible. The sword of truth is the only way to pierce the denial and start moving forward out of the darkness.

Getting grounded in the truth

Our world is a collective reflection of our individual choices. If we want to heal the world, we need to start within ourselves. This starts by getting grounded in the truth.

I find it helpful to question my perspectives and motives, consistently and honestly, to check in with myself. This is part of my daily mental ninja work, to keep myself unsubscribed from the early life programming that taught me to pretend it's okay when it's not and to go along to get along.

This practice is also excellent for building immunity to gaslighting, manipulation, propaganda, and other forms of suggestion or coercion that we are exposed to by other people, the media, social media, and through advertising and entertainment. The more the virtual world advances, the more of a challenge it will be to stay grounded in the truth and the more diligent we'll need to be with our self-honesty work.

This is a self-care sobriety practice that you can apply to almost anything. Ask yourself:

- Why am I doing this?
- Why do I believe this?
- What purpose is this serving in my life?
- Where does this perspective come from?

Be sure that you're taking an objective look at the answers and not indulging in fantasy, illusions, lies, or rationalizations. When we have addictions, we will rationalize and lie to ourselves to hide the pain. That's where the addiction lives—under the lies and on top of the pain.

Sometimes addictions involve physical substances. Other addictions are more about an escape into fantasy, feelings, illusions, or ideas. Those are the trickiest ones to identify because their very existence is invisible.

Addictions are often layered in a web of lies. The invisible addictions are usually the ones that cause our deepest inner conflicts and mental blocks, which keep us stuck and unable to liberate ourselves and move forward to the next level.

If you're able to identify an addiction that you're still struggling to let go of, ask yourself:

- Where is the lie?
- Which stories are you telling yourself to justify why the addiction is okay and necessary?
- What is the pain that you're trying to escape or avoid?
- Where in your life are you committed to, accepting, or participating in something that's not okay for you?

We often lie to ourselves to avoid facing a painful truth. It's normal to want to deny the ugly truth to avoid the pain. However, in order to create a better life, we must first be willing to admit the truth so we can move through the denial and come out on the other side.

When you're using GPS, it needs to know where you are so you can get to where you want to be. If we aren't honest with ourselves about where we are, then we are not going to be able to go where we want to in life. That includes all levels from the individual to society.

As we align more with the truth, the body and mind will detox from the lies, illusions, distortions, fantasies, pretending, and denial. Lying and pretending makes us sick over time. This is why we are living in a sick society. The purer and truer your body and mind are, the quicker you'll feel sick when you start lying to yourself or pretending.

It's like when you consistently eat healthily and then introduce some junk food into your system. You're going to feel acutely awful for hours or even days after eating that. Yet someone who eats junk food regularly doesn't feel that because her body has become desensitized to the consistent toxicity.

The same is true with the energy we ingest from contact with other people. When you've detoxed your life of emotional manipulators, as soon as someone toxic shows up, you'll notice very quickly. It will be a visceral experience. But if you keep toxic people around and another one shows up, you might not notice how you feel around that person since you're desensitized to the toxicity.

When you hang out with people with whom you can't be honest and authentic, those relationships will inevitably turn toxic, even if everyone involved has good intentions. Inauthenticity leads to unsustainable relationships. When you sacrifice truth and authenticity for connection, that means you're abandoning yourself and not meeting your own needs. This usually comes from childhood programming.

If you have to pretend to be someone you're not, or to like something that you don't like, or if you have to silence yourself and not speak about things that are important to you because the other person would think you're crazy or get angry at you, then that's not a healthy connection. Everyone involved could have good intentions, but these are not the kind of relationships that can survive the truth.

Your authenticity is your truth about who you really are. When you're living truthfully with yourself and someone shows up pretending to be something he's not, you will notice the dissonance. You might not know exactly what the lie is, but you will feel the space where the absence of truth exists. And vice versa.

If you want to make a breakthrough into liberation, make the commitment to be more honest with yourself about the choices you make daily. That includes the thoughts you allow to take seed in your mind, the people you allow in your life, the projects you participate in, and the actions that you create in the world.

Consider the consequences of your choices. Is that really what you want in your life, or is it what someone else wants or told you that you should want or do? Is the choice coming from you, or is it a conditioned behavioral response coming from automaton programming? You can be compassionate with yourself while also being honest.

If you want to shift away from the pretenses, I highly recommend you take a break from social media, especially Instagram and Facebook. I haven't used those platforms in a few years now and it's like having a new nervous system. Of course, I had to completely rebuild my self-worth internally after I released the addiction to external validation. It was challenging, but worth it!

If you take a few weeks off and then go back to those platforms, you'll probably notice exactly what I'm talking about. You might feel disgusted and anxious just scrolling through the feed a bit.

If you're like most people, you probably have an addiction to using those platforms. I used to, and I was in denial. I rationalized that it's fine because *everyone else is doing it*. Canadian author and motivational speaker Bob Proctor wisely said that if everyone is going a certain way, you should probably consider going another way.

If there are relationships and situations in your life that you're not sure about, you can give yourself some space to feel and process your feelings. With the distance, you'll likely gain clarity about whether it aligns with your authenticity and belongs in your life, or not.

Sometimes we have to make space to get a new perspective of the truth and to figure out if a relationship, habit, or situation is really aligned with who we are and where we are going. Give yourself permission to create the space to allow the truth to enter. You will gain new insights.

Integrating the shadow

The transmutation of the shadow into light is an alchemical process. It starts when we can meet our shadow with compassion, acceptance, and truth instead of rejection, denial, or avoidance.

The shadow is where we find all the vulnerable parts that we want to deny, suppress, or not see. These are the parts that weren't seen, loved, heard, or valued by others. The shadow is what we are ashamed of, the parts that were shamed by others and the parts that tell us we aren't enough or that something is wrong with us.

The shadow gives rise to the false self. These are the protector parts that hide the shame, the ones that make us feel safe, but hidden behind a mask. The false self projects judgment, hatred, and disdain onto our true self (and others) when it's scared.

The false self exists so that we can fit in, be accepted, gain approval, and stay connected—though it often sabotages connection as well. It's rooted in childhood experiences. It helped us to feel safe as kids.

However, the suppression of the shadow disables our authenticity, individuation, and uniqueness as well as our ability to be honest with ourselves and others.

We can observe the shadow through the human body, behavior, and autonomic processes. Shadow work is the process of self-awareness and integration of these parts.

Due to the shame surrounding the shadow, it can be helpful to face it with curiosity, compassion, and non-judgment. It starts by honestly noticing the signs that indicate when you're in your false self:

Which automatic behaviors belong to the false self?

Which thoughts belong to the false self?

Which fears belong to the false self?

What are the needs and desires of the false self?

Which qualities, interests, and truths do you suppress to fit in with your family or peers?

The point of this self-inquiry is not to beat yourself up. First, validate that the false self was the intelligent response to survive and feel safe when you were a kid. That includes *in utero*, when you became energetically imprinted with all your mother's thoughts, emotions, and experiences of her environment, which came from her unresolved trauma.

It can be extremely valuable to take this exploration to the next level:

How did the false self's behaviors, thoughts, needs, and desires serve you in childhood and adolescence?

How is it serving you now?

What is it costing you now?

We each have an individual shadow. There's also an ancestral and collective shadow, based on what has been denied, unwanted, unseen, unheard, devalued, suppressed, and repressed in a family, culture, or society.

As we integrate our individual shadow, we upgrade portions of the ancestral and collective shadow, too. Every aspect of our inner work of transmuting the darkness into light brings a beneficial contribution to the world around us.

When you're willing to see the parts of yourself that you didn't want to see, the vulnerability of that honesty initiates a breakthrough and metaphysical healing process leading you toward liberation.

On the other hand, you'll notice that when you aren't being truthful with yourself, you get stuck in mental blocks, frustrations, and conflicts. You keep externalizing it all and blaming others, which causes you to feel victimized and powerless. That obstructs your freedom and forward movement.

Admitting the truth is not the same as healing. If only it were that easy! It won't be that easy for society either.

We need to talk about what happened and be honest with ourselves about how each of us participated in it. It's directly related to our unresolved childhood and ancestral traumas. Understanding what happened is important. Yet simply focusing on the external truth will not move us forward through the liberation and integration process.

Being truthful with ourselves is the start of liberation and healing.

CHAPTER 12

LIBERATION

The Way Out

Captivity is a state of consciousness that will endure and continue to be triggered repetitively by life experiences until we transform the underlying patterns holding that perception in place.

Many of these distortion patterns are rooted in childhood and what we inherited from our ancestors. Our world has also been socially engineered to make us forget who we really are, to outsource our power and worthiness to someone or something else.

Liberation is a process of *remembering that we were always free*. Our consciousness is more powerful than any abuser, control system, or dark forces. We have been programmed and tricked into believing otherwise.

The way out of the state of captivity and into true liberation means more than just leaving the abusive relationship or situation. At that point we're still trapped in the darkness, living in the enslavement of injustice.

We end up unknowingly perpetuating that state of disempowerment when we don't recognize how our thoughts about the injustice can lock us into an identity, a frequency, a story, a path where more injustice happens and so we continue to find supporting evidence that we are victims of life.

We are free and we always have been. The captivity is the distortion, corruption, and program. The matrix is set up to invite us into that state of disempowerment, enticing us to stay in the perception of enslavement after we've been abused. Then the frequency of captivity reverberates back from the universe and life brings more of those experiences.

Until we root out the deeper patterns that are holding the construct of captivity in place, we will continue in a state of powerlessness. That dysfunctional dynamic could go on indefinitely, passed on to the next generations who learn *that's just life*.

This chapter explores liberation from the state of captivity as well as the surprising fifth parameter that makes it challenging to step into freedom.

Common myths of liberation

These are some very common false assumptions about liberation after abuse, crimes against humanity, and other forms of relational harm. Most people think that they'll miraculously feel free when certain things happen:

- When the truth comes out,
- When the perpetrators are in jail,
- When the perpetrators are dead, or
- When you go no contact with the perpetrators and their enablers.

However, none of these actually leads to liberation.

Perpetrators often dose their victims with *hopium*, a form of false hope, which is also known as the anesthesia of the masses. This leaves people comfortably numb waiting for disclosure, hoping that the truth will one day be revealed by a hero and then all will be well because we will all be free. The truth can be relieving and validating, however it doesn't heal us simply to know the truth.

While it would be great to see accountability for the injustices committed, that doesn't resolve the deeper issues that will continue even if all the perpetrators are in jail.

Even if we do get justice in the court system, that's not the same as healing. It would feel validating and relieving at first so it could be easy to confuse that as healing. But after the initial relief wears off, you'll notice that the hole in your heart is still there because that's not true liberation.

The dilemma of justice

Abuse, deception, betrayal, and other forms of relational harm leave people wanting revenge. It's normal to have those thoughts and feelings. It's not okay to act on it.

It's also important to distinguish between revenge and justice. Revenge is about getting even and making others feel the pain that you feel. That will inevitably lead to more pain and perpetuating the spiritual war because such actions carry a karmic burden, which entraps you further into the darkness. Leaning into revenge can be tempting, yet it's a dangerous path.

Sometimes revenge is referred to as reactive abuse, or offending from the victim position, when the victim harms the perpetrator in reaction to the abuse and harm that was done. But that's also how a victim can become a perpetrator. "He made me do it" is never an excuse for harming someone. In fact, that's what most abusers say. Be careful when fighting the darkness that you don't cross over to the other side.

Justice is about an external validation that harm was done, and it involves some kind of legal or social solution to balance the scales. In an ideal world, there would be justice in these cases. But as we've already explored in this book, abusers don't take accountability for their actions and it's the enablers who maintain the abusive system by doing the bidding of abusers and tyrants in order to make themselves feel safe. This is why we rarely see justice coming from the human world.

Of the thousands of stories I've heard over the years about abusive relationships, families, and workplaces, only a very small amount of the victims ever got justice in the legal system or in their social system. For the most part, the perpetrators keep getting away with it and other people keep enabling it. Understandably, that can create a strong attachment to injustice.

Without closure from the perpetrators, most abuse victims end up having to create an inner sense of closure. Otherwise, they become stuck indefinitely in injustice and captivity.

Sometimes miraculous things happen, bringing justice to injustice. I would call this poetic justice. Nothing goes by in this universe without the inevitability of divine justice, though we don't always get to witness it. It's rarely on the timeline that we want because it's on divine timing.

At a soul level we already know this and can find peace in remembering this cosmic law of cause and effect. It's the ego that wants to see justice now because it's attached to the story of injustice. The ego believes it won't be okay until there's justice. This is another trap that keeps people in a state of captivity. In fact, I'd assert that this is the fifth parameter, which only becomes visible after a person wakes up to the abuse and tyranny. Awakening is not liberation. The awareness of the injustice activates a trip wire.

What I often see among people recovering from abuse is that they are so focused on the injustice that they can't heal or move on without closure through justice. They get stuck in endless rumination about what happened and how unfair it was. They're not wrong. But, unfortunately, in those cases, it's like the abuser won—not just because he escaped justice, but also because the victim is living in captivity, even long after leaving the abusive relationship or situation. The darkness prevails.

A person who escapes an abuser or abusive system isn't necessarily free. If you're still fighting with the abuser in your mind, unable to heal and paralyzed from moving forward or enjoying life, that's not liberation. That's a prison cell with holographic bars.

Freedom is not just about escaping the physical environment of abuse. Liberation is a state of consciousness. True liberation is when you can create closure for yourself by releasing the layers of pain and heavy feelings caused by the injustice so that you can reclaim your joy. This first requires a perspective shift, which the ego is going to resist initially.

While trying to help people to empower themselves, I realized that the biggest challenge after the awakening is the attachment to the injustice. That's what keeps a person stuck in the powerlessness of victim consciousness. I am very familiar with that predicament because that's how I drifted through most of my life. I didn't fully understand this until going back in the trenches during the early 2020s.

Letter to a victim

I lived full time in the victim state of consciousness for almost thirty-eight years. I didn't realize that I could be right about the injustice *and* release my emotional attachment to it, so that I could start to create the life I wanted to live, free and liberated from the past.

During those years, I was constantly ruminating about all the injustices done to me and those thoughts made me feel really bad. There was no justice in any of those experiences—they just got away with it. So, I became increasingly more resentful because the feeling of injustice was building every time it recurred.

That kind of thinking and the corresponding feelings were creating an energetic vibe that I was putting out to the universe: "I am a person to whom injustice happens." And, so, life gave me more situations and people causing injustice because those were the energetic instructions I was (unknowingly) giving the Law of Assumption.

What we assume about ourselves is mirrored back to us. It's not a judgment or punishment—it's more like cause and effect. I wanted to be right about the injustice more than I wanted to heal. My ego was *really* attached to that. I thought that liberation meant I would get justice and then I could let it go.

Life sucked in the powerlessness of the victim consciousness. It was miserable—like a self-imposed prison uniquely tailored for me, mirroring all my fears, insecurities, and resentments. I didn't realize *I was both the captor and the captive.*

That was how the abusers kept abusing me even long after I left those situations. I was fumbling around in the darkness. My holding on to the emotional and mental attachment to the injustice meant they kept winning because they still had control over me. I couldn't see how I was the one maintaining that reality.

That's the state of captivity. It's an internal state of consciousness. That's why it doesn't have to be physical confinement. Perception is reality.

I was free to move about, but I wasn't free in my soul. I was tethered to the negative feelings of the injustice against me, and so the world around me was tainted in those dark colors. If someone had told me that back then, while also offering compassion for what I'd been through, maybe I could have saved myself a lot of time and suffering. Or maybe my ego would have been defensive and doubled down on wanting to be right. We aren't always ready to hear the truth.

After the victimization, the darkness leaves a piece of itself in the person it touches. The battle turns inward and it's like we're fighting ourselves. We have the free will to release ourselves from the state of captivity at any time, yet the emotional attachment to the injustice isn't so easy to give up. It has a strong gravitational pull.

It's understandable because the injustice isn't fair. Yet the only way to reclaim our power after such experiences is to set down the bag of heavy feelings. We can only do that once we've released the emotional attachment to it.

One of the wildest things I've seen in my life is the incredible poetic justice that inevitably occurs when a person stops carrying the burden of those heavy feelings for the perpetrator. It returns energetically to the rightful owner in divine timing, and that usually doesn't take too long.

So, you have a choice once you've awakened to the abuse and tyranny in your life and in our world: Will you stay stuck here in the emotional attachment to the injustice, unable to move forward? How much longer will you put your liberation process on hold while waiting for justice? As long as we are carrying the heavy burden for the perpetrators, they keep getting away with it. It's a dirty trick!

This is a very tough dilemma. It's painful to accept that there might not be justice for the crimes that were committed and the harm that was done. In an ideal world, the perpetrators would meet justice in the courts. Yet this might not happen, at least not immediately, because our court systems are so corrupt.

Perhaps we will be fortunate on planet Earth that eventually attorneys, judges, and other international players with conscience will bring about some kind of legal justice for the crimes committed against humanity. There have already been some of these little victories such as the Queensland Supreme Court ruling in 2024 that COVID vax mandates for police officers and paramedics were unlawful and failed to adequately consider the human rights implications.[72] Yet somehow they rationalized that it didn't mean *all* vax mandates were unlawful. In April 2025, Idaho became the first state in America to create protections for personal medical autonomy with the Idaho Medical Freedom Act ensuring that Idahoans "will never again be compelled to undergo unwanted medical interventions as a condition of employment, education, or daily life."[73] Schools, institutions, state government entities and businesses will be prohibited from denying access, services, transportation, or opportunities by discriminating against individuals' medical choices. Yet so far, these victories of justice are rare and of limited scope.

We will not find liberation by simply focusing on the perpetrators and what they did. While understanding the truth about what happened is a very important part of the early stage of the journey, it will not lead to healing unless we do the inner work. The good news is that we don't have to depend on external sources of justice in order to liberate ourselves.

Empowerment and liberation will not be found through achieving justice. It will also not be found through a rescue fantasy or a savior. No one is coming to liberate us. We can save ourselves from captivity by choosing to release ourselves from the obligation of carrying the burden of pain for those who harmed us.

The gravitational pull of victimhood

In the early stages of recovery after abuse, it often feels like things will never get better, that healing isn't possible, that you're not capable of making it any better, and that good things don't happen for you in life.

There's so much in our world that's out of our control. You have no control over what others do. You can't control what the global mafia do. You can't control the economy. You can't control the war. You can't control the government.

So, what can you control?

That's an empowering question to ask yourself. The only thing you have control over is your perspective and how you respond to life. Your choices are where you'll find your power. Your actions and choices matter. You matter. Your choices are creating your legacy.

When everything feels out of control, come back to center and ask yourself where in your life you're not taking responsibility where you could be. In what ways are you giving away your power to external people and circumstances?

When you're in the victim state of consciousness and hear the word self-responsibility, you'll interpret it as blame. If someone encourages you to take responsibility for your own choices and participation in life, you might even call him a victim blamer. That's when you know you're in a state of captivity.

When people patronize and pander to victims, they often encourage a victim-superiority stance by telling them they're better than the abuser. They stroke their ego with titles like *empath*, saying that the only reason the abuser preyed on them is because they're so empathic, unlike the abuser.

While it's true that the victim could be empathic and good, this simplistic explanation isn't the whole truth. Without embracing the greater nuance of the truth, this perspective merely serves the ego and keeps a person stuck in victimhood. The false power of superiority inevitably flips into inferiority as these are two sides of the same coin.

It's not easy to admit that when you're in a victim state of consciousness. Yet when you're ready to liberate yourself, you'll be able to accept that you can be right about what happened *and* heal from it.

In the victim mindset, everything is black and white, so nuance is inaccessible. In a state of empowerment, you can recognize the power and responsibility of your choices in terms of how you're participating in your life *and* acknowledge that what other people did wasn't your fault.

If you're not there yet, it's okay. Maybe you're still trying to learn something from the state of powerlessness. Or maybe you're starting to realize that there's another way to live beyond captivity. You just didn't know how. You didn't see any other possibility than the reality you were living because that's all you knew. I was there, too, and there is a way out.

It's far easier to keep blaming someone else for your feelings or your life circumstances—whether that's your family, your ex, your boss, your neighbor, the government, or the global mafia. But the external focus and the attachment to the injustice will keep you stuck in the powerlessness of captivity, living a miserable life.

One of my clients described the feeling of victimhood like a heavy coat that's always covering her. I told her that's good news! The amazing thing is that you can take a coat off because *it's just a f*cking coat!* She said that was the best line ever. Something about that realization was the perspective she needed to reach escape velocity, to overcome the gravitational pull of victimhood, and shift her state of consciousness toward liberation.

The first threshold

Many people live a lifetime in the state of victimhood, never realizing what happened to them, never recognizing their own power, and therefore never moving beyond that point in the journey. That becomes the ancestral burden that gets passed down again and again and that's why humans are born into this matrix of trauma, captivity, and powerlessness.

Once we realize what happened, the first level of new awareness after abuse is almost entirely external. This is when people recognize the atrocities committed and the harm done to them by another person or people. At this point the victims usually develop a ravenous hunger to learn everything they can about the abuse as well as the red flags of abusers. They start learning the lingo and finally have the words to describe what happened to them. Then they need to be able to tell their story to an empathic witness who believes them and listens.

This is the most common point where people get stuck. Realizing they were victimized, it can be tempting to remain indefinitely in the obsession and rumination about what happened. When that happens, the person is unable to move forward through the healing process. The vast majority of people watching content online about narcissistic abuse, and most of those who woke up to the tyranny in our world, are not liberated. They're still in this phase, focused externally.

There's a very clear threshold between the first two stages of healing. I call it commitment to self-responsibility. This is the moment when people have a sudden realization of how they have been participating in the dysfunctional dynamic of their life and relationships.

When we can recognize that we were reacting to life from automatic programming instead of making free choices, that's a powerful breakthrough. It's the awakening from the insanity of doing the same thing and expecting different results. The state of captivity begins to dissolve when we realize that our choices are where we find our power. Then we can reclaim sovereignty and autonomy over ourselves through this commitment to self-responsibility.

That's a tough truth to embrace because it means being honest with ourselves. It's also incredibly empowering, because when we take responsibility for our choices, we start to own our power.

Then we can enter the next stage of healing, which is about strengthening our empowerment. This is where we have the opportunity to start making new choices because we have new awareness. And when we make new choices, we get new results. That's when the deep inner work begins.

The way out

True freedom isn't just leaving the abuser or abusive situation. It's about releasing the heavy burden and integrating the wisdom of the past so you can create a new future.

It will require first facing the external truth and then the internal truth. When you finally have the visceral realization that you're the one holding yourself captive, you'll see that it's just an illusion that you were conditioned to believe is real. You can have compassion for yourself *and* liberate yourself.

The lowest state of consciousness is that of the powerless victim, frozen and imprisoned in the past. This is what the perpetrators taught you and convinced you is real. That's where the global abusers aim to keep humanity because, in such a state, we are easy to control.

What do you need to face *inside* yourself in order to restore your power?

Victimhood is a stage, not a life sentence. It's a state of consciousness, not an identity. Things can get much, much better as we do the inner work of self-healing and actualization.

Your liberation is a process of deliverance that happens as a result of your cumulative choices. It will take some time, but happens naturally as you work your way through the layers of constraints holding the perception of captivity in place.

Along the way, keep reminding yourself that you are free. Freedom is your human birthright. People taught you to believe otherwise because other people taught them the same thing. We have all internalized lies from family, friends, intimate partners, bosses, politicians, media, culture, social media, and other sources, both spiritual and human, as well as the way we interpreted those events and what that meant about us.

No matter how stuck you might feel right now, there is liberty from the bondage. Deliverance from the prison of darkness is possible even though it may not feel like that during moments of intensity and overwhelm. The perception feels real. And that's why liberation from captivity starts with a perspective shift and then a new commitment to taking 100 percent responsibility for your life and choices.

A big part of self-responsibility involves continually working on self-regulation to increase your inner power. That means regulating your emotions so you can respond—instead of reacting—to people and life. This will help you to build inner security instead of looking for someone or something external to make you feel safe, validated, distracted, or calm.

One level of self-regulation could be self-soothing. Let's differentiate this from the old addictions and escapisms that we explored in Chapter 4. Self-soothing is a healthier coping mechanism than the old ways of escaping reality. Self-soothing is calming and relaxing, but it's a *temporary* relief and doesn't transform the underlying defensive patterns that keep us in the primal state of captivity.

For example, self-soothing activities that calm anxiety could be listening to Solfeggio frequencies or binaural beats, meditating, doing yoga, journaling, running, walking, or working out.

The next level of self-regulation means doing inner work and digging deeper when you feel triggered.

A trigger is like a breadcrumb calling your awareness to a pattern in your life. As you get to the bottom of your triggers, you can empower yourself by identifying their origins and resolving the past, layer by layer, so they no longer have control over you in the present.

When you learn how to master the art of self-regulation, you can approach your triggers with curiosity and compassion instead of resistance and suffering. When we can create space between the stimulus and response, we open up the possibility of accessing and downloading insights, intuition, creativity, and other forms of new consciousness instead of the same old automatic reaction.

The more you clear emotional attachments to the past, the more liberated you'll feel, the more energy you'll have, and the less reactive you'll be to things that trigger your traumatic memories. The past becomes neutralized and that's when it reveals deeper gifts. Putting self-regulation into practice consistently will help you to unlock your power and liberate yourself from captivity a little more each day.

As we clear up our resentments and regrets, things start to feel *much* lighter, and we free up energy for intuition, healing, and growth. We usually don't realize how heavy this stuff is until it's not there anymore. During the process, the emotional attachment to injustice starts to dissolve on its own because it has nothing to stick to anymore.

The best way to release each of the resentments caused by injustice is to first meet it with compassion and curiosity instead of judgment. Then identify how each resentment served you, albeit in a distorted way. For example, sometimes resentment feels like protection from something, or permission to set boundaries and keep ourselves safe.

Likewise, with the regrets; you'll want to approach yourself with compassion, curiosity, and non-judgment. Then identify how the regret served you. Sometimes we don't realize we are holding on to regret as a form of self-punishment or motivation to not make the same mistake again.

Once you understand how it served you, you can identify what you learned from each resentment or regret. This part is about the integration of the knowledge, strength, wisdom, and other virtues that we can extract from the pain. Our challenging experiences transmute into exquisite gems for the soul's evolution.

Once you figure out the benefit and learning that came through the resentments and regrets, and you have the inner desire to release these, then you can decide how you want to learn instead. For example, you might prefer to learn those virtues through inspiration, love, and grace.

As we clear the resentments and regrets, the heavy feelings dissolve. When we stop carrying that energetic burden for those who caused the injustice, it is returned to its rightful owner in divine timing, and poetic justice will be served.

Liberation is possible and it's an inside job. There's no external person, event, or circumstance that can set us free. We are already free. Everything else is just a program of perception.

What gives you a sense of freedom and power? It's something that feels effortless. When you're doing it, you're filled with passion and confidence. Notice what freedom and power feel like in your body when you're doing that, so you can start to connect more with it.

For me, it's dancing. No plan, no choreography, nothing in particular. It's just letting go and allowing my body to move spontaneously. When I'm dancing, sometimes I forget that I'm moving my body. That's when it's most effortless because it's just pure freedom.

I'm safe. I'm sovereign. I'm free.

CHAPTER 13

FINDING ALLIES

Restoring Trust

Many people have lost friends and loved ones in the 2020s due to the increasing chaos taking place in our world and how it polarized us to take a stance one way or another.

This has left most of us wondering how to restore trust in relationships, families, communities, and society. Trust is essential for social connection.

But much like in abusive families, workplaces, and other social groups, restoring trust isn't easy due to the dysfunctional system dynamics and the choices that individuals in the system are making to maintain the status quo.

The system is designed to defend the system.

Social systems are complex relational dynamics between individuals that create a whole. Each individual has the potential to affect the system, yet the collective status quo of the system often overpowers a person's will to go against the grain.

This is why abusive families and other social systems don't suddenly change when one person wakes up and calls out the abuse. When you take that brave stance, the system will turn on you. That usually means you'll need to find allies outside your social system whom you can trust and share reality with.

This is also why the biggest challenge after relational trauma is the damage to trust. How can you trust people who are still denying reality, acting like everything is fine?

If they haven't had a reckoning, they're just one fear campaign away from doing it again, or worse. We can only move forward together when trust is restored; otherwise it's going to be a repetition of the past.

How do we restore trust and move forward if we are living in such vastly different reality paradigms that have led to the collapse of trust in our relationships and society?

It starts with finding allies

We don't respect ourselves when we keep trusting a person who has broken the trust in a relationship and not taken accountability or action to repair the damage. Without accountability, there is no path for rebuilding trust.

When trust is broken in relationships, you could stay and volunteer to continue being a victim of ongoing transgressions, or you could choose to empower yourself by setting boundaries and no longer extending trust to those who have proven to be untrustworthy.

In January 2022, a Rasmussen poll revealed some incredible statistics:

> Nearly half (48%) of Democratic voters think federal and state governments should be able to fine or imprison individuals who publicly question the efficacy of the existing COVID-19 vaccines on social media, television, radio, or in online or digital publications. Only 27% of all voters—including just 14% of Republicans and 18% of unaffiliated voters—favor criminal punishment of vaccine critics.
>
> Forty-five percent (45%) of Democrats would favor governments requiring citizens to temporarily live in

> designated facilities or locations if they refuse to get a COVID-19 vaccine. Such a policy would be opposed by a strong majority (71%) of all voters, with 78% of Republicans and 64% of unaffiliated voters saying they would Strongly Oppose putting the unvaccinated in "designated facilities."
>
> While about two-thirds (66%) of likely voters would be against governments using digital devices to track unvaccinated people to ensure that they are quarantined or socially distancing from others, 47% of Democrats favor a government tracking program for those who won't get the COVID-19 vaccine.
>
> How far are Democrats willing to go in punishing the unvaccinated? Twenty-nine percent (29%) of Democratic voters would support temporarily removing parents' custody of their children if parents refuse to take the COVID-19 vaccine. That's much more than twice the level of support in the rest of the electorate—seven percent (7%) of Republicans and 11% of unaffiliated voters—for such a policy.[74]

Knowing this, how can we find common ground? Have they changed their minds, or are they simply no longer being publicly encouraged to be vocal about their dehumanizing ideology?

The terrible irony is that many of the same people who virtue signal with slogans like *just be kind* were also advocating the segregation of certain groups of people from society. How many public apologies were issued for this? Very, very few.

Likewise, how do you trust someone who knows you were abused by another family member, but keeps talking about how wonderful that abusive person is?

Forgiveness is an important part of the later healing process in order to cultivate a deep sense of inner peace. However, this does not imply reconciling the relationship with a person who hasn't repented for his transgressions. It would be foolish to reconcile relationships where trust has not been restored because the breach of trust will inevitably happen again.

Forgiveness is a release of the inner tension blocking the restoration of joy and love. It's often anti-climatic, as it happens naturally after releasing the resentments and obligation of carrying the bag of heavy feelings for a person who caused the injustice. It has nothing to do with trusting or uniting with people who wish you harm or did you harm.

On an interpersonal level, you could choose to end such a relationship to protect yourself from further frustrations, loss, betrayal, and harm. Yet it's a tough call when it's your loved ones. It's perhaps even more challenging in society at large.

Trusting another person is like making an investment in his future behavior. While we all have the potential to evolve, if a person hasn't taken accountability and made those changes explicitly, it's wise to take into consideration that past behavior is usually the best predictor of future behavior.

Sometimes we make good investments of trust and other times we suffer losses. When we realize we've made a poor investment, the best option is usually to cut our losses and pull out before more loss and harm is incurred.

A relationship becomes dysfunctional when trust is absent. So does a family or society.

When trust collapses, social cohesion disintegrates, and people no longer want to work together because that would mean trusting those who have shown themselves to be untrustworthy. What's interesting is that people on both sides of that trust wound can have distrust of the other, albeit for different reasons. Who is right? That depends on whom you ask.

The absence of trust also entices people to look for false gurus and saviors who make promises of safety and unity, which leads to more harm. The trust wound increases like compounded interest over time as the debt keeps rising.

So, what can we do amidst the collapse of trust in the global system, in workplaces, in families, communities, or other social groups?

Leaving a social system without accountability, and finding allies outside that social system, is usually the ideal approach, albeit challenging. This is ever more complicated in a global society.

Our human history has plenty of examples of the collapse of trust, yet there's something unique about our time now. In the past, the so-called enemy during wars and other historical turning points was usually an outsider.

Nowadays that division goes straight through the hearth and home. A family unit is the root of a society. The ax of polarization has split all the way down to the roots this time. Admittedly, the social engineers have done a spectacular job of getting us to go along with the divide-and-conquer approach by provoking our fears and distorted desires, just as any skilled perpetrator does in an abusive relationship or family.

In a war-torn climate of distrust, from the micro level to the macro level, the restoring of social trust starts by finding allies.

How do you find allies?

When I worked in narcissistic abuse recovery, I often used the phrase *own your reality*. This means to define reality from your perspective. Get clear about what's real and what's important to you.

Of course, you should be willing to re-evaluate and adjust your perspective when reality changes or new information becomes available. Yet you also need to recognize when you're being gaslit and should not allow someone else to distort your perception of reality, even if many people see it that way and there's only one of you. A collective trance is *very* contagious.

Speak the truth with courage. Give yourself permission to be more candid. Be willing to listen, too. When we don't speak our own bias about how we see reality and what matters to us, we won't be able to use that as a filter to find alignment with others.

It can be scary to speak so honestly due to the fear of rejection, upsetting someone else, or turning someone off. Yet that leads to delaying the inevitable, often wasting a lot of time in the process. You can only sacrifice your authenticity for so long until you start losing yourself trying to maintain a relationship or situation.

In speaking the truth, you'll quickly identify who your allies are and who are not. Don't waste your time trying to convince people to see the world the way you do. Speak to those who want to hear what you say, to those who want to add to the conversation instead of running from it or attacking you over it.

During COVID, I would try to start the conversation with people. Sometimes I saw horrified faces and backed off. Other times people yelled at me and called me names, so I walked away. But in a small percentage of those conversations people responded like they had just found water in the desert. They were thirsty for that kind of conversation, and perhaps too afraid to speak first.

Using the truth as a filter, you'll increase the likelihood of finding those who resonate with what you have to say. Yes, of course, you'll have some unpleasant experiences, but finding out sooner rather than later will save you much time. Choose your allies wisely.

It's also important to recognize that just because someone sees something in a similar way doesn't mean that he's your close ally.

This is true for a person escaping an abusive family system or workplace as well as at the societal level. Many people learn this lesson in support groups for abuse survivors, or by contacting another ex of their ex, just as many learned this during the COVID abuse. The enemy of your enemy is not always your friend.

Our personal and professional relationships will be our greatest assets, or worst liabilities, during the increasing instability in our world.

Since the early 2020s, many people have been questioning where they belong in terms of their geographic location, friendships, workplace, colleagues, intimate relationships, and even family. This has been one of the greatest gifts that the challenges brought. It's an opportunity to re-evaluate and choose aligned social connections where you will thrive.

Speaking the truth shows you where you belong and where you do not. This act of courage reveals the truth, and lies, surrounding you. Sometimes you might choose to end certain relationships due to their influence in your life. Other times people will pull away from you, or push you away, because the truth you're speaking feels threatening to their perception of reality.

When you're truthful with yourself and others you will find more aligned relationships and turn away from the toxic ones, or even those that simply aren't a match of core values and direction. Living in authenticity, truth, and accountability helps you to find your people and build trust on a solid foundation.

Redefining your inner circle

Choosing your inner circle consciously is very important for protecting your sense of peace, wellbeing, health, wealth, and joy.

Notice who the people are with whom you share the most time and energy. This could be in person, on the phone, or even online. As the saying goes, *you become like the people you surround yourself with, so choose carefully*.

Pause right now and write down their names. Ask yourself why you like hanging out with them, what kind of characteristics they have that you admire, and what impact they have on your life. This exercise will open your eyes to something you didn't see before.

If you realize that their impact is not positive, that you don't like who you are when they're around and you don't want to become like them, then move those people to the periphery by reducing contact.

In some cases, you might choose to remove people from your life completely if they're a toxic influence, even family members. You're allowed to do that! Give yourself permission to honor your experience, free from the obligation of making someone else comfortable or happy.

The restructuring of your inner circle is a way of owning that space responsibly, giving your time and energy mainly to those who are closest to you. That investment brings a return, whether positive or negative.

The most dangerous part about being in contact with toxic people is the temptation to subscribe to their reality, whether that's their worldview, their opinions about who you are and what's possible for you, or their own negative self-concept that is projected onto you when they get triggered by your success, health, happiness, or confidence.

As you do the inventory of your inner circle, ask yourself if the people you hang out with are draining your physical, psychological, and spiritual wellbeing or if they're supportive and inspiring.

How do you know the difference?

Notice how you feel when you think about them. Notice how you feel when you're with them and then afterward. Give them a particular text tone on your phone and notice how you feel when you hear that tone. It could be especially helpful to journal those insights so you can track them over time.

Be careful that you're not accepting toxic, draining people in your life simply because you're afraid to be alone. It's much better to be alone for a period of time so you can focus your energy on taking care of yourself and healing from the past. Then you can reset and attract people on a different level. You may want to hire professionals or seek out mentors who can guide and support you through such a challenging time so you're not entirely alone.

It will not benefit you to keep feeding people who are sucking the energy from you, re-traumatizing you, and setting you back, leaving you with little to invest in your health, happiness, and dreams. You're not helping them either, that's just enabling.

Toxic dynamics will keep you stuck in the negative cycles and replaying the trust wound. This implies recognizing your own participation in the dynamic. That's the only way to make new choices and attract new relational experiences in your life. Otherwise, you'll move those people out, and keep finding more of the same and wondering why.

When you have mutually supportive people in your inner circle who are living in a similar reality, it's much easier to stay unsubscribed from the abuse narrative and speak the truth. Your allies help to keep you sane in a world of insanity. It's nearly impossible to start moving forward in the healing journey after abuse and tyranny without these kinds of allies.

The most valuable commodity in a social system

It's interesting to see the parallels of trust in the monetary system, which is based on the value and velocity of money and trust in interpersonal relationships, family, and society, which are based on the value and velocity of virtues like honesty, trust, communication, and attunement.

As the global system of trust is collapsing, that's a cumulative result of what has been happening on the interpersonal and intrapersonal level between and within individuals.

The breakdown of trust at the micro level has become so normalized that the shocking events in our world aren't alarming to much of society. Many people have become so accustomed and desensitized to betrayal, lies, and corruption that they look the other way, perhaps hoping it gets better without any action of their own. Denial doesn't lead to self-trust or the building of trust in relationships.

Our personal integrity and the quality of relationships we choose (intimate partnerships, friendships, community, family, business partners) will determine how we move through the challenging times ahead. The same is true for a person escaping an abusive relationship, family, or workplace.

In ideal relationships, all parties contribute something of value to the others. Everyone has the opportunity to thrive more than he could alone.

In the rarest and most beautiful types of relationships, additional layers of exchange lead to greater healing, emotional maturity, spiritual development, motivation, inspiration for learning, prosperity, depth of meaning and purpose, as well as a shared mission in the world.

Trust is the glue that holds healthy relationships together. It improves the quality of life.

The cliché, "Love is all you need," is a lie.

Have you ever loved someone who betrayed you, abused you, used you, or didn't value you? Trust—not love—is the foundation of relationships. Trust is where love grows, and when it's destroyed, the whole thing collapses.

Trust can be powerful and strong, yet it's also fragile. Trust is built slowly over time, and it can be destroyed in an instant. When divergent values or agendas emerge and a debt of trust occurs in relationships, war breaks out there, too.

Once trust collapses, there's nothing left but an empty abyss between people.

Sometimes people try to keep making it work, pretending everything is okay. It's tempting to think that love is enough to keep it all together. But over time, the emptiness grows and the love rots into hatred through doubts, suspicions, painful memories, resentments, regrets, jealousy, anger, and even paranoia.

Have you ever stayed with someone after she cheated on you or betrayed you in some way? Probably not a day went by that you weren't thinking she could do it again. And she probably did.

Sometimes people choose to grow and change, but that requires inner work, self-awareness, self-honesty, self-responsibility, and the humility to admit to and repair mistakes. Not everyone is willing to venture into the territory of self-healing and personal evolution because it's not the easy path.

The relationships we choose will either lead to a frustrating and painful repetition of past stories, or they will be an opportunity for a more positive form of mutual growth and healing, the creation of a new future.

One way or another, we learn the most about ourselves through the mirror of our relationships, a perspective we can't often see in solitude. Our relationships have the power to elevate us or destroy us.

Everything depends on the trust factor.

It's the same in society. As we watch layer after layer of the chaos unfolding in the world, we are each being shown the areas where we could heal and expand our self-trust based on our response to what's happening. That will change the level of trust in our relationships.

Undoubtedly, we all have the opportunity to learn and grow through this process. It's much easier when we have trustworthy allies at our side.

The frozen past in a relationship or society

When we are triggered and emotionally provoked to hyper-react, that means there's something unresolved from the past to heal.

Where we are numb and shut down, unable to really feel what's happening, that means there's something even *bigger* and unresolved hidden beneath the surface.

Thomas Hübl, an Austrian mystic and collective trauma-healing facilitator, teaches the importance of recognizing the mute pain in trauma—the *absencing* or numbness. In his training programs, he teaches that what's really hurt is silent and frozen. The thing that's hardest to find has the highest healing impact.

People talk about many problems in society, yet what we aren't really talking about is *exactly* what would help us to heal the most. The same could probably be said for most relationships.

Valuable wisdom is frozen in the trauma of the past. It is stored in the subconscious energy field as well as the nervous system and body, from the tissues all the way down to the DNA.

When we are unable to feel and witness the pain in ourselves and in the world, we are unable to access the information that can lead to learning, healing, and growth.

What we are unable to feel in ourselves, we cannot feel in another person or in the world. And vice versa.

Trauma recovery at the individual level involves the inner witnessing of feelings that emerge, as well as processing the emotional residue of the past that has been frozen, fragmented, and exiled.

The same is true at the collective level of trauma in society. Somewhere in our collective consciousness is the frozen, unintegrated trauma and wisdom of our ancestors who survived difficult times before. Likewise, that's where we will find that of our time.

Thomas Hübl describes the trauma frozen in the body like ice, and our awareness like the sunlight that restores movement to the water. Hübl also describes the mutual witnessing that can take place between two people in a relationship, as well as in a society through healing communities, as part of the relational repair.

When we don't feel each other through the attunement of our nervous systems, then we are unable to truly connect or feel emotionally safe. We can feel misunderstood, unmet, or unseen. Then we get defensive. Trust cannot grow there.

When trust is broken, the relational repair takes place through rebuilding a foundation of truth and safety.

Our ability to be in tune with others only exists when we are present, authentic, and not triggered into defense mechanisms.

Our defensive reactions (fight, flight, freeze, and fawn) come from the unprocessed fear and pain of the past. These become our maladaptive relational dynamics, which cause disconnection, dysfunction, and distrust between people instead of connection.

When the autonomic nervous system perceives danger, whether that danger is real or perceived based on past experiences, it triggers the brain to react according to the default survival programming of the past, moving us from a state of social connection into defensiveness. Essentially, it takes us from the present into the past. Every time this happens, the past keeps repeating and there's no real future.

Trust involves *presencing* with one's self and others. This is the backbone of all relationships. The best way to cultivate presence is by integrating the past so we can truly be here now with awareness. We'll explore this inner work of building resilience in Chapter 17.

The origin of trust in social connection

Attunement is a form of mutual witnessing that creates empathic resonance between people. It's about having awareness of, and responding to, another person's emotions. This process is the foundation of building trust in relationships.

It's a form of energetic communication that doesn't require words but sensing at a deeper level. It often happens (or does not happen) without our conscious awareness. We feel it (or the lack of it), often without understanding what exactly we are sensing.

When a baby feels the mother feeling the baby (imagine an infinity symbol), the baby experiences a sense of safety and connection, which is imprinted in the nervous system as a default program of secure emotional attachment. The baby feels seen, heard, and held.

A mother whose nervous system is overloaded with her own fears, anxiety, undigested experiences, and unresolved traumas won't be able to be present to share this attunement with her baby. Instead, she will transmit her stress to the baby's neurological system, which becomes the default program of an insecure emotional attachment. The same thing likely happened to her, as the patterns repeat ancestral trauma loops.

Without awareness, a mother will use the baby to soothe her own pain. In these cases, when the baby cannot trust that the mother will notice or meet his needs, the baby's nervous system is programmed to feel chronically unsafe and disconnected.

Our childhood and ancestral pain become the obstacle to trust in our adult relationships. However, when we process and integrate our traumas, we can reprogram our defense mechanisms and nervous system to create new opportunities for attunement, safety, trust, and connection.

When trust collapses beyond repair

When trust breaks down in relationships it's because one or both parties have produced something that subtracted value from the relationship instead of adding to it.

The question is: Can trust be repaired after it collapses?

Sometimes it might be a minor breach of trust that can be repaired through communication, accountability, and restorative behavior. These minor losses of trust and safety could be the result of a mistake due to ignorance, a misunderstanding, or a missed opportunity for attunement (a blind spot) where one person was unable to feel the other and maybe vice versa.

Other times it could be much bigger damage to trust due to a transgression. Without honest, direct communication and accountability, there can be no relational repair. Words need to be put into action so that the trust can be rebuilt on something real, not just an admission of fault, an empty promise, or a *potential* for change.

In our post-2020 world, trust has been destroyed between people, as well as between We the People and our corrupt governments, media, corporations, medical systems, civil institutions, and global organizations.

More people are realizing that we've been lied to, deceived, misled, silenced, coerced, and in some cases even injured or forced to comply with something that violates our personal values. These were not mere mistakes. It was intentional harm, and the biggest breach of trust was the claim that it was *for our own good.*

We the People have also lost trust amongst ourselves. We are becoming acutely aware of everyone's true values based on how we responded to the events unfolding. As trust continues to collapse, we are learning whom we can really trust and whom we cannot, both in our personal lives and in society.

Many people are wondering which personal and societal relationships can be repaired and if it is even possible to restore trust where it was so badly damaged.

In any kind of interpersonal relationship, when two people have opposing values, that will inevitably lead to betrayal due to the conflict and incompatibility of values.

When one person values liberty and another person values the perceived safety of control via tyranny, each will act according to his or her values and both will feel betrayed in some way. Trust will be left in a state of irreparability because both parties will experience transgressions against their personal values. With diametrically opposing values, it's very difficult—if not impossible—to restore trust.

This is why it's so very important to have allies.

Of course, we will never agree entirely about everything with everyone or anyone in the world. People are free to have their own perceptions and values, as long as they're not taking harmful action toward another person or that person's property. When that golden rule is betrayed in a family, workplace, social group, or society, there's usually no common ground on which to rebuild a foundation of trust.

The only option at that point is to seek out allies where trust can be built, forming small communities and networks of people who share common values and live in integrity with those. Even where we disagree, we can honor and respect one another's right to life and liberty.

The path of restoration

The path to repairing and restoring trust involves returning to the truth. This step is essential and cannot be bypassed if the structure of the relationship or system is to be built on a solid foundation.

This hasn't happened in society, and, so far, it doesn't appear to be possible anytime in the near future. We are ever more polarized, and that is a global problem reflected in local nuances.

We can't even agree on what the truth and reality is. We are also realizing that we have incompatible values. This would be the moment to get a divorce based on irreconcilable differences in marriage.

But how does that work in society?

For the most part, we have no idea of the whole truth about what happened and what's really going on now, with the exception of some evidence that has seeped out of the festering boil in the dregs of society, which appears ready to explode at any moment. For example, the Johns Hopkins study cited in Chapter 10 that revealed that lockdowns did more harm than good. There is increasing evidence presented by embalmers around the world, of strange clot formations they're discovering in people who have died in the recent years.[75] It's finally being acknowledged in medical studies that thrombosis is one of the side effects of the vax.[76] Myocarditis has been recognized as another severe side effect, especially in young men.[77]

There is still much more that we don't know and may never find out. Denial, suppression, evasion, and obfuscation will not lead to the restoration of truth and trust in the world, in families, or in relationships.

This current trajectory is not leading to social cohesion; in fact, just the opposite. It appears we are at an impasse in society. At that point, the only way to restore truth and trust starts within oneself and builds through gathering allies of kindred spirits and minds in small communities and networks.

Many people feel that it's challenging to gain a sense of community. Maybe you have a loneliness wound from childhood caused by abuse, emotional neglect, betrayal, loss, rejection, or abandonment. The old pain is often amplified through social experiences that trigger these same feelings.

One of the most common stories I hear from people is that as kids they felt alone and scared because their parents were always fighting. They wanted to fix it but felt powerless to do anything about it. These kinds of experiences can lead a person to have low self-esteem and feel like they're not good enough or they don't deserve to have mutually supportive relationships in their life. We'll explore the importance of doing inner-child integration work in Chapter 15.

The amazing thing is that every time we have a new positive social experience, the new energetic imprint overrides the old ones. We access new levels of thriving through community, which we cannot do alone or with those who reinforce old wounds.

OLD IMPRINT

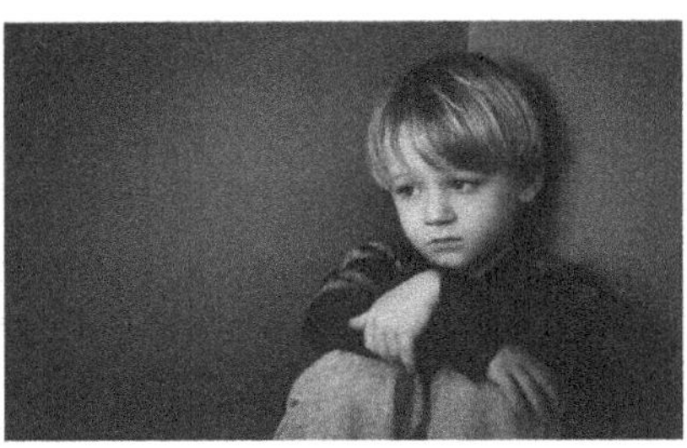

NEW IMPRINT

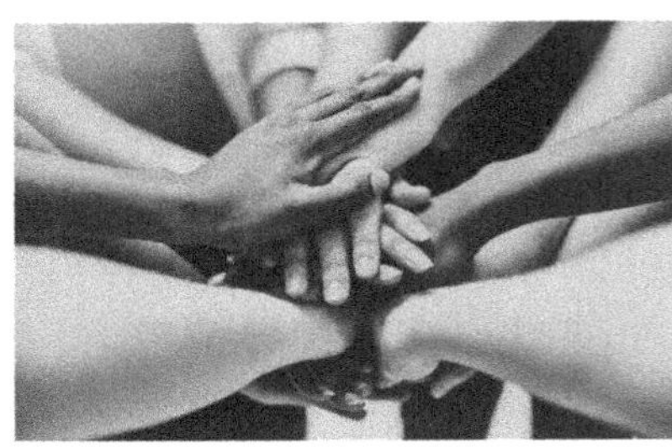

Optimizing your ability to connect with allies

- Encourage and contribute direct, transparent, honest, and sincere communication in your relationships.
- Ask questions for clarification when things are ambiguous or vague.

- Be curious and compassionate when approaching communication. Instead of assuming why someone does or believes something, ask him or her to elaborate.
- Don't allow misunderstandings to fester with your loved ones. If you don't talk about it, that will create distance as well as bigger confusion and distortions.
- Offer the gift of presence to yourself and others. Use your breath to consciously bring your awareness down from your head and into your body. Breathe. Listen. Feel. Notice what's there with curiosity and compassion.
- Make eye contact with others and notice who they are with curiosity instead of expectation and assumptions.
- Make a conscious effort to avoid distractions when you're spending time with yourself in solitude or with your friends and other loved ones. That means: Put your phone away!
- Take some time daily, preferably outdoors in nature, to connect with your Creator as if you were talking with a friend. Build an honest connection with your Creator and remember that this is an important ally.
- Take an inventory of your priorities. We are all busy. Are you prioritizing time and energy for what (and who) really matters to you? Do your priorities reflect your core values or are you drifting from what most matters to you?
- Give yourself permission to have standards and set boundaries with other people. Your boundaries are first and foremost with yourself. Be willing to disappoint or upset people who don't like your boundaries. Honor your values and standards.
- Have faith that good people exist and that it's possible for you to find aligned relationships. Don't allow past betrayals to make you bitter and resentful.
- Strike up a conversation with people in public who feel approachable. Be open to learning something. You will.
- Speak the truth more often. It can be scary to risk rejection, but it will save you much time and disappointment when you explicitly share your perspectives with others. You'll find out

very quickly who your allies are and who are not! You'll also build courage in the process.

CHAPTER 14

SELF-WORTH

Your Greatest Immunity

One of the most important foundations for healing and developing immunity to abuse is rebuilding self-worth. This is about strengthening your inner sense of worthiness, which is your divine birthright.

We live in a world where it's all too easy to fall into the lie of unworthiness. We are conditioned and programmed, in increasing ways through technology and social media, to seek external validation to prove our worth.

There has never been a more important time to build self-worth than now. We are constantly being assaulted by propaganda and social engineering that aims to convince us we need to qualify our worth through something external, such as social status, money, beauty, or social media vanity metrics.

In an unparalleled devaluation of our inherent worth as human beings, during COVID, we were told that there are "essential" workers, implying that the rest of us are non-essential, meaning worthless.

Shocking as it was to hear that, it was just the prelude to the AI revolution when many jobs will soon become obsolete. That will leave many "useless people," as philosopher and advisor to the World Economic Foundation, Yuval Harari, has often said in interviews. In a 2017 video clip, Harari asks, "How will they find some sense of meaning in life when they are meaningless, worthless?"[78] He suggested the answer is a combination of video games and drugs.

No doubt our world will continue to change rapidly. A foundation of self-worth will help you to keep adapting and finding solid ground no matter the chaos going on around you and no matter how much the external world is trying to trick you into believing you're not worthy.

The key to self-worth is the *self* part. True worth cannot come from outside. We are constantly bombarded with messaging that's trying to convince us that we aren't enough, then provided with solutions to fill that void. But none of that works. The search for worth outside the self leads to an inevitable crash because it's not coming from within. Everything external can be taken away at any moment.

Your inner sense of worth is your divine birthright and no one can take that from you unless you allow it. Your innate worth is a gift from the Creator. God willed you to exist. You have the right to exist, and you are worthy of existing.

Everything an abuser does has the aim of making the target feel unworthy of basic human dignity. It may seem so obvious that this is based on a lie. Yet when you're in it, the slowly escalating and insidious acts to tear down your sense of worthiness can happen faster than you think.

If you've been through abusive relationships or subscribed to any of the societal narratives that you're not good enough because you're not this or that, then you're likely struggling to restore your self-worth to factory settings.

One of the best investments you can make in your self-worth is to get off social media platforms. The algorithm is programmed to target men and women differently based on all the demographic and behavioral data it gathers from phone and online habits, which you consented to by accepting the "Terms and Conditions." Remember: The dark forces always tell us what they're doing.

Notice how you feel when you cruise through the feed on the social media platforms you use. What kinds of thoughts are you hearing in your mind? How do you feel about yourself after using social media? Are you using it to fill the existential void and suppress feelings?

The aim of the darkness is to make you believe that you're not enough or that something is wrong with you. These are lies. But when you believe you're unworthy of the most basic human dignity, you'll likely make agreements with those campaigns and comply with anti-life measures, accepting the further degradation of your body, mind, and spirit. This is why your self-worth is a powerful tool for building immunity to abuse and spiritual warfare.

The restoration of self-worth

The opposite of self-worth is shame. Shame is a spiritual agreement that collapses and immobilizes us, causing us to hide or self-sabotage. It's identity focused. Shame isn't about what you did (or didn't do)—it attacks *who you are*. It can make you feel worthless, unlovable, or defective. Shame leads us away from our true self and into the false self.

Shame is different than guilt. Guilt says, "I did something bad." Shame says, "I am bad."

Guilt is behavior focused. We feel guilt in response to actions we've taken (or not taken). You'll likely feel guilty when you've acted against your values and betrayed your own integrity or hurt someone. Guilt is part of a healthy conscience. It's meant to keep us on track and to encourage repair when we've messed up.

Shame becomes a weaponizing force used to gain compliance, whether in an abusive family system, workplace, or society. John Bradshaw described this in his book *Reclaiming Virtue: How We Can Develop the Moral Intelligence to Do the Right Thing at the Right Time for the Right Reason*. He said the culture of obedience is "the kind of morality that produced the Nazi Holocaust," when people "remain naive and unconscious in the face of such evils."[79]

Bradshaw was wise to recognize that the main root of violence in a community or society is violence at home, particularly the abuse and neglect of children. He described it as *the death of their spirit rather than their bodies.* That kind of upbringing produces kids who will likely grow up to be vulnerable to ideological violence.

People who carry shame from childhood abuse and neglect will inevitably have impaired ego development due to how it distorts the sense of self. Bradshaw recognized how this kind of childhood programming sets people up to become easily recruited into cultures of obedience where all kinds of abuse, discrimination, and violence are possible due to their tolerance of it. It's the same reason why people fall into toxic relationships. *It feels like home.*

Bradshaw was ahead of his time. This is an incisive explanation for why so many people easily become enablers of the types of societal abuse we saw during the COVID campaign. People reported their neighbors for violating arbitrary COVID rules, and wanted to segregate others from society for not complying with the measures. Parents went along with the physical isolation of their kids, interrupting and stunting important developmental processes. People condoned the elder abuse that took place in care homes and hospitals. People dehumanized and segregated those who didn't take the shots. In other words, people were devaluing the basic human dignity of those they believed to be less worthy. The enablers became weapons by proxy of the ideological violence.

Inferiority and superiority are two sides of the same coin that flip back and forth. Likewise, when we feel shame when we are down, we will feel grandiosity or pride when we are up. Superiority, pride, and grandiosity can convince us that we are righteous, and that blind spot can easily lead to ideological violence.

Bradshaw's reflections on the societal implications of shame are incredibly relevant to what happens in abusive social systems and relationships. He contemplated the virtue necessary to know how to respond in such circumstances, "when sure knowing is lacking but our conscience or our circumstances demand that we act."[80]

This was indeed where we all found ourselves in 2020. While it was difficult to know what was really true amidst so much propaganda and censorship, *something felt off*, and this challenge called on us to listen to our conscience.

Bradshaw said that Aristotle called that virtue *phronesis*, which means moral wisdom in Greek. Aquinas translated it as *prudentia*, which means prudence.

Bradshaw recognized decades ago that we urgently need the virtue of prudence in our world. He advocated prudence, describing it as *conscience in action*. "Prudence is our situational conscience, or conscience as applied in the unique, concrete situation a person is facing."[81]

This definition of prudence as situational conscience implies nuance. It's not about having rigid rules and ideology but about applying our conscience in each unique situation that arises in life. It's exactly what we tapped into during the COVID campaign when we didn't consent to lowering our worth for not complying with tyranny disguised as *for the greater good* or *for our own good*.

It can be vital for anyone who has experienced abuse, use, neglect, or mistreatment to conduct an autopsy of past relationships and other situations where those kinds of shame-based experiences occurred. What effect did that relationship or situation have on your self-worth? How did you restore your worth after outsourcing it to others?

I would recommend you do a similar self-reflection exercise on how you've responded to the tyranny of the 2020s, regardless of whether you took the shots and complied with the other measures. This isn't about blaming, shaming, or judging. It's about self-awareness—and these insights will be very valuable in the future. What impact did your decisions have on your self-worth? How did the virtue of prudence show up in your actions? How could you embody more prudence in your daily life?

You can do a journaling exploration of those topics to highlight areas where your self-worth could be rebuilt. It would be helpful to process the resentments and regrets that you may still have as a result of those experiences, as well as any residual fear, guilt, or shame. This review and release can help you to make better and braver decisions next time.

You could undertake a similar self-reflection on how you were affected by childhood experiences at home and with your peers. Was there shame caused by abuse or neglect at home, or bullying at school?

What impact did those early life experiences have on the formation of your self-worth and sense of self? Are you still defining yourself in some ways based on your early life programming and how others treated you?

Restoring self-worth through inner examination

Abuse results in the crushing of self-worth. It degrades you to the point that you start to believe you don't deserve your most basic human rights, such as the right to say no.

Do you believe you're allowed to define your values and protect these? If not, you can start by visualizing that it's possible to say no and that you're allowed to do so. You are allowed to give yourself permission to uphold your values, even when others disagree. You don't need to convince anyone else, either.

You'll know you still have low self-worth when you have a strong inner critic, when you frequently hear self-blame, self-judgment, and harshness toward yourself in your inner dialogue. When we are harsh with ourselves, our heart is closed in a stance of self-protection. Then we feel walled off and separated from others, which further exacerbates the feeling of shame like a self-fulfilling prophecy.

You may also notice some self-pity and false guilt, which are related to low self-worth. You might observe that you unknowingly internalized the pain and projections of others. That probably helped you to feel safe as a child, but now it's distorting your self-perception.

What other people do *to* us can cause resentment that bothers us for a long time. If you were aware of the abuse taking place during the COVID campaign, you probably have resentment toward the perpetrators as well as toward enablers, such as family, friends, or even humanity as whole for how they were accomplices to the tyranny. I've had to work through this resentment in recent years as well.

If you process the resentment, you'll be able to release that burden before it turns into bitterness, tainting your life with that shade. How did the resentment serve you? Is it still serving you?

Whether you reconcile certain relationships or not, that's your choice. Be sure you're evaluating honestly what effect those relationships are having on your self-worth today, not based on the past or a fantasy of the future. It's challenging to feel worthy when you surround yourself with people who don't see your worth, yet you consider them your *loved ones.*

When we fail to honor ourselves, those regrets can be the heaviest burden because we know we participated in lowering our own self-worth. If you complied with abuse or tyranny, you'll have regrets to process.

It's important to first recognize why you did it. Probably it was to survive and feel safe, to maintain a job or relationship, or to keep your family together. You'll want to work through those layers so you can release yourself from this burden before it turns into self-hatred, causing you to abuse yourself and continually replay the past.

The more honest and compassionate you are with yourself, the more effective this work will be for you. The more of the emotional residue you release, the lighter and freer you'll feel.

When you're observing your inner dialogue, you might notice the subconscious belief programs that keep you undervaluing yourself and settling for less than you're worth. What do you say about yourself in your self-talk and out loud to others? When did you first learn to talk to yourself that way? It probably goes back to childhood.

For each of the painful experiences that are still bothering you, what did you make it mean about you? What's the story you tell yourself about who you are based on what happened?

How would your life change if you had healthier self-worth?

What's the cost of not having self-worth?

What would be the cost of having healthier self-worth? Would it mean leaving a relationship, or letting go of certain friends or situations in your life?

What would you have to start saying no to in order to raise your self-worth?

The filtration system to build self-worth

To rebuild your self-worth, you'll need to identify what really matters to you in life. These are your personal core values.

Then you'll need to set standards and boundaries to protect them. In the process of setting new boundaries that protect what matters to you, you're naturally raising your self-worth.

What most matters to you? And what does that look like in real life?

You can do a values exploration to see what's important to you. Then you'll know what you need to protect with your boundaries, thoughts, and actions. Knowing your values will help you to determine what you want to say yes and no to.

Not everyone has the same values. Values are personal beliefs. Clearly identifying and knowing your values is a necessary step for protecting what matters to you. If you don't know what's important to you, you won't know what to protect when it matters most.

The practice of setting standards and boundaries to protect what's important strengthens your self-worth, which is an important protection against the corruption of evil forces, whether human or supernatural.

Why is self-worth your greatest immunity to mistreatment and misalignment? It filters out the toxic people and misaligned situations pretty quickly. While some manipulators are super covert and not easy to recognize right away, as soon as you do see the signs, your self-worth, standards, and boundaries will provide you with a system for disengaging and protecting what most matters to you.

When you're in doubt about how to respond to a person or life circumstances, your self-worth will remind you to honor your dignity before responding. One of the best ways you can build dignity is to work on self-regulating your triggers so you can choose your response consciously and own your power of choice instead of reacting emotionally when you're dysregulated.

Setting boundaries to rebuild self-worth

Saying no is usually the first boundary people learn to set when they've lived a lifetime unaware of their right to have boundaries due to childhood programming.

People who have accomplished great things have often said that successful people say no most of the time. In which areas of your life do you want to have more success? That will help you to figure out where you need to start saying no more often.

But before we can have boundaries, we must set our standards. A standard is a *yes*. It's what you *do* want. It's important to set standards for yourself in terms of how you show up in your life, the kinds of projects and situations you want to be a part of, and the kinds of treatment you'll accept from others.

Once you have standards, then you can create your boundaries. A boundary is a *no*. It's what you *don't* want. A boundary is a line you draw to protect what matters to you.

Integrity is a result of alignment between your values and your actions. This implies having standards and boundaries. Do you live your daily life by taking action that's in alignment with your values? Where do you currently need more alignment in order to step into greater integrity?

If you don't know whether to say yes or no to an invitation in the moment, you might be in a freeze state. This means you'll have a delayed reaction. It's very common after childhood trauma. If you're unsure, don't force yourself to give an answer just to make the other person happy or satisfied. You can say, "Let me get back to you soon on that." Take some time to reflect and respond later when you have clarity.

Are there any areas of your life, or particular relationships, where you're currently sacrificing your integrity or authenticity? If so, take an inventory of those relationships and situations to see how you can bring in more of the authentic you in order to get in alignment. Perhaps you need more boundaries. In some cases, you might choose to walk away to maintain your authenticity and integrity.

Give yourself permission to disappoint people with your boundaries. Sometimes people will be upset that you won't do what they want. You are not responsible for how they feel. You are responsible for protecting what matters to you.

Healthy self-worth means that you are willing to invest in long-term peace over a temporary perception of peace. Be willing to say no and tolerate the disappointment or anger of people when they don't get what they want from you. You don't have to internalize that.

Likewise, it also means being willing to say no to yourself and delaying gratification for the long-term investment in your value. Your boundaries are first and foremost with yourself.

Are there any projects, relationships, or situations you're participating in that go against your values and lead you away from your goals? Take an inventory of those so you can determine ways of integrating your values more and aligning your life with your goals. If that's not possible, ask yourself why you're still investing in those projects, relationships, and situations. How is it serving you?

It's also important to recognize false self-worth, which is external and superficial. This is based on a dependence on external validation or posturing, masking, acting tough, or feeling better than others. Are there any ways in which you're using external validation to hide insecurities?

Upgrading your identity based on self-worth

Visualize yourself with genuinely high self-worth. Who are you when you know your worth? How do you respond to people and life in that state?

It's important to practice this visualization so you know what it feels like to live in worthiness. This is a way of retraining your subconscious based on the upgrades you're making to your sense of self.

What would you need to give up to step into that future version of you? These could be particular habits, vices, relationships, projects, belief systems, or thoughts.

Remember, no one else can take away your self-worth. Your self-worth is your divine birthright. It is not something you earn or have to prove. *It is who you are.* Your worth is based on how you define it. When your definition of worth is the same as the Creator's, you'll truly understand what worthy means. You can ask God to download you with the highest definition of worth from God's perspective.

If you're in a state of captivity, you probably don't believe that you're worthy. Maybe worthiness sounds impossible to you right now because you've never known what it feels like to be worthy. You might be wondering, when you're on the floor, how do you get back up so you can start to reinvent yourself?

If you have zero self-worth, initially, you might need to find something that you do believe is worth getting back up for. For some people, that's their kids, grandkids, God, life purpose, family, or legacy. This is your *why*—but it's not the *source* of your self-worth.

Once you have a reason to get back up, something bigger than yourself that you believe is worth fighting for, then you can start to redirect your self-worth work internally.

While it can feel impossible to shift out of such a state of consciousness—the shame of learned helplessness—remember that we can do seemingly impossible things. Think of a mother who lifts a car off the ground to save her child. You can rebuild your self-worth.

I want to remind you that human potential is infinite. It can be used for good or for evil. This is our free will, our free choice.

If you want to believe that you have worth, act in ways that reinforce this belief in yourself. When you make a mistake, don't beat yourself up about it, adding to the shame. Come back to compassion. You can be honest with yourself *and* not shame yourself for what you did. Recognize why you did it and how it served you. Identify where that program came from and ask yourself if it's still serving you, or if you want to change it by making a new commitment.

When you stray from your standards, return to integrity as soon as possible by returning to your values and boundaries. Through reflection, you can recognize where you took a turn down a divergent path so you can make new aligned choices in the future.

The restoration of self-worth is a work in progress. Keep upgrading your identity of worth as you learn, heal, and evolve. You'll see along the way how robust your immunity has become when it's easy to turn away from invitations to degrade your own worth.

CHAPTER 15

GROWING UP

How Did It Serve You?

By the time all things COVID happened in 2020, I had already done a lot of self-healing work over the prior two decades. I thought I was living my best life but, very quickly, I found myself slipping into self-destructive habits.

The global trauma was bringing to the surface my unresolved past. I went back into the victimhood consciousness. The injustice of what was brewing in the world was stirring to the surface a familiar feeling.

I saw the overt and covert abuse, particularly the emotional manipulation happening around the world via the fear bombardment. I saw how the parameters for Stockholm syndrome were being laid out. I recognized the anti-life program of self-sacrifice disguised as *for the greater good.*

I knew where that was going, because the same cult programming happens in abusive families, workplaces, and other social groups. If you don't consent to sacrificing yourself, they sacrifice you. A covert abusive system programs you to destroy yourself before others destroy you. The act of self-sacrifice is a distorted way of feeling some control over a powerless, hopeless situation. It can feel like the safer thing to do.

Initially I felt paralyzed by an inner conflict because I knew I needed to speak up, but I was stuck in fear surfacing from the past. There weren't many people taking a brave stance, so it was easy to be targeted. I knew I was going to lose a lot if I spoke publicly about the abuse. My livelihood was at risk. The part that I really didn't want to admit was that my ego was also on the line. The decision to honor my conscience in the face of tyranny would later come with the confrontation of my blind spot.

As I was watching it happen in real time, I observed myself struggling with the superimposed unresolved childhood trauma that I didn't realize was still there. A big blind spot started revealing itself to me, which would take the next years to unravel and process before I could shift back to empowerment and integrate more of the past. Eventually I was able to see how it all served me and how my experiences could serve others.

Before 2020, I didn't realize that I had rebuilt my self-worth on false grounds. It's not *self*-worth if you're gaining a sense of worth through external validation, which was exactly what I was doing on social media platforms. The vanity metrics of likes, comments, and subscribers soothed my ego and gave me a false sense of having healed from my past trauma. It was a *distraction* from the pain. It also gave me a false sense of belonging, connection, and significance.

I didn't realize I had disordered desires, as Dante Alighieri would say. I was chasing after the wrong things and avoiding the pain of emptiness and loneliness—remnants of the unresolved past—through seeking external validation.

Admitting to myself that I had created a false sense of self-worth through the social media presence I'd built was inevitably going to lead to an ego death. I also knew I didn't want to keep creating on those platforms, which was not something I had foreseen. In 2020, using social media became like voluntarily entering into an abusive relationship with all the censorship, gaslighting, and shadow banning, as well as the smear campaigns from people online.

I knew I needed to let the old system collapse, yet I felt paralyzed by the inner conflict between my conscience and my primal brain. The fear was winning. Initially, I wasn't ready to face the reality of what I was going to lose, so I engaged in self-sabotage. It was a decision I made, though it doesn't feel like you're choosing it when you're on default subconscious mode. It's automatic.

The choice is made without your awareness when you're in a primal state. That's why self-sabotage happens relatively quickly, and before you know it, you're looking back wondering how you got to that point.

I spent most of those days doom scrolling and imagining where it was all going. I became hyper-focused on what *they* were doing to us, much like I had years before when I was voraciously researching narcissists, psychopaths, and other abusive characters. I was obsessed with what *they* had done to me because I was in a state of victim consciousness.

I forgot that's not where my power is.

I thought I had already learned that lesson. But unhealed layers of that pattern got triggered and rose to the surface in a new circumstance with the events unfolding around the world.

The externally focused victim consciousness would linger with me for the next few years. I kept focusing on what *they* were doing, using that as an excuse to not take 100 percent responsibility for my life and my choices. I was reacting, instead of being proactive in my response to life.

A core part of my pre-2020 message was about empowerment through self-responsibility in the recovery process, but I got pulled back into the state of captivity. Apparently, I had to return to the trenches to understand it more deeply, then transmute more of my own darkness into light.

It was a rough time, but it was also a gift. It gave me the opportunity to gather more wisdom, to suffer, and to connect with my own humanity, so that I could transform the learning into compassion for my personal evolution and the service I offer others who are on a similar journey of liberation and empowerment. It was time for me to grow up and move to the next level. This is our opportunity as individuals, families, communities, and society as we move through these challenging times.

Unresolved childhood trauma and the 2020s

It blows my mind how many people don't know that they have unresolved childhood trauma. It's quite similar to how most people are acting like nothing happened in the early 2020s. Most people would rather not deal with it, so they suppress it or find something to distract or escape from it. It's not a judgment or a blame. It just is what it is. And I get it—I was there, too.

I've also noticed something like a mental firewall that prevents us from honoring our experience of childhood because that implicates our parents. Many people are afraid to say anything that's less than completely positive about their parents. Deep down, the wounded inner child is still afraid of punishment. Yet in silence, the dysfunction, pain, and suffering keep going, generation after generation, like a curse. It takes courage to face the truth and end the cycle.

We can honor the truth about what happened and how it affected us without blaming our parents. While parents are responsible for what they do to their children, they, too, made decisions that don't feel like real choices because they were running on automatic subconscious programming. How many generations ago did the dysfunctional patterns start? It's hard to say who is at fault because traumatized people usually traumatize their children unknowingly. The constructive perspective is about responsibility, not blame.

When we discover that we've been abused or neglected, the first phase of recovery involves identifying and naming what happened. This is incredibly relieving because people finally discover that they're not crazy, there's nothing wrong with them, and it's not their fault. It's normal to create distance from those who hurt you so you can heal.

Unfortunately, though, most people confuse that initial discovery with empowerment. The path to healing isn't about the ability to make character judgments and recognize the red flags, though that is important for setting boundaries and no longer tolerating abuse. Healing is about ending the cycle by doing the inner work.

When people tell me "I had a great childhood!" that's often a sign of emotional neglect that they don't recognize yet. With a little digging, the patterns usually reveal themselves and people start to understand how their early life programming and ancestral trauma continue to repeat through less-than-ideal circumstances and relationships.

Things start making more sense with new awareness. Yet the point isn't to get stuck here in the awareness of why we keep responding to life in similar ways, but to use that awareness as inspiration to start to make new choices. This is where we find our power.

Denial is a powerful yet primitive survival mechanism. It serves the purpose of helping us to survive intensely stressful experiences like childhood trauma or any kind of trauma in adulthood, including the trauma intensification happening on a global level since 2020.

Denial becomes maladaptive when, as adults, we are blinded to our participation in our present circumstances and therefore rendered powerless to do anything to make them better. True power comes through responsibility.

I often ask people, "How did your life change since 2020?" Most tell me something mundane like they broke up with their significant other, they moved, or they switched jobs. Like it was any other year.

How is it that people don't remember when the whole world shut down? Every aspect of human life was about COVID that year. You couldn't even open a marketing email from a corporation without reading about what it was doing differently "due to COVID."

It boggles my mind that people don't remember the intense fear bombardment and forced isolation, how their movement was restricted, when families and friendships were divided and conquered, when people were segregated from society and threatened by public officials if they didn't submit to medical procedures or devices. Not to mention all the other insane things that were happening, as I described in Part One.

You may have heard of abuse amnesia, where a person can forget the memories of abuse that took place. That's the brain's way of adapting to an abusive relationship or situation so a person can keep enduring it when it feels inescapable. It's a lot like denial.

This survival mechanism now affects many people after what has happened since 2020. It's the same thing that blocks people from remembering childhood traumas or from perceiving events as traumatic because it just feels like life. Most people don't recognize how their maladaptive behaviors were programmed by trauma.

It's fascinating to observe how we responded to the post-2020 trauma in a very similar way as we responded to our childhood trauma. This isn't about blaming, shaming, or judgment. It's about having curiosity and compassion to understand *why we do what we do*. Without that awareness, we are powerless to change our behavior.

Many people were in complete denial about the abuse trauma taking place during the COVID tyranny. Many of them still are, despite all the revelations of evidence since then. Denial was probably how they learned to feel safe in childhood. Yet it carries a heavy price over the long term because the trauma keeps compounding. The stress in the world triggered our primal survival mechanisms of denial and defense. These are automatic programs that we aren't aware of until we can finally see our patterns.

Some people responded to the COVID threat by fighting. That was likely how they created a sense of safety in childhood. We've seen so much fighting, anger, and aggression online and in real life in families, between friends, and among complete strangers since 2020.

Sometimes people fight to maintain the illusion of a happy family or what they want to believe about their parents. That usually involves fighting those who try to point out the truth about abuse, neglect, alcoholism, addiction, or other harm. Some kids got thrown on the streets as young teenagers and they learned to fight to survive. Some might have learned to fight against abusive authority figures in their family or against enablers who didn't see, or acknowledge, the abuse that was taking place.

Others responded to the COVID threat by fleeing into addictions and distractions like alcohol, drugs, food, porn, shopping, gambling, video games, fantasy, or workaholism. Flight was their way of creating safety in a stressful and unsafe environment in childhood. Of course, the particular substances and activities will often differ from childhood to adulthood, but the underlying defense mechanism is the same. That's why we've seen addictions skyrocketing since 2020.

Another way that people coped with the COVID threat was by freezing. The freeze response is when a person shuts down and collapses, which is something many childhood trauma survivors did to feel safe. The body also shuts down vital systems like respiration, heart rate, and digestion. We can't stay in that state long without dying, so as humans when we feel like we can't escape our stressful circumstances, we adapt by dissociating or otherwise fleeing reality. In Chapter 3, we explored how common this has become in the post-2020 world.

Over time, the dissociation becomes a functional freeze state where people often binge-watch TV and videos or scroll on the phone and social media consuming mindless content. When we're overwhelmed and zoned out, we shut down. That means we're not present and we lose track of time. This often leads to losing track of days, weeks, months, and even years. Procrastination and apathy set in, which makes it challenging to get mobilized.

Others responded to the post-2020 trauma by fawning and complying, whether they knew something wasn't right about what was happening, or not. In childhood, they learned that the easiest way to survive the lack of safety in a seemingly inescapable situation was to people please—to perform and prove their worth, doing what the parent, caretaker or other authority figure wanted. Going along for the ride brought a temporary reprieve from the abuse or emotional neglect. Yet, as we explored earlier in this book, compliance doesn't end the abuse. It leads to a loss of dignity and self.

About 80 percent of the world complied to some degree with the control measures from 2020 to 2022. Some were injured, harmed, or killed in the process. The long-term psychological, neurological, physiological, and spiritual consequences are ongoing, while the authorities continue to gaslight us and many people are continuing to gaslight themselves by pretending like nothing happened, or that what happened was necessary.

Of course we can all use a combination of the "fight, flight, freeze, and fawn" defense-and-denial reactions depending on the moment or situation. From my observations, we usually have two primary survival mechanisms. Identifying these with curiosity and compassion is very helpful for upgrading our programming. First, we must understand how these defense mechanisms helped us to feel safe and survive. Then we can recognize how these same habits are sabotaging what we really want in life.

From what I've observed, people who have been actively working on healing their childhood trauma, at some point since 2020 started using these experiences as an opportunity to dig deeper.

As the triggers come up, we have the possibility to notice the similarities between the present and the past, and to clear more layers of the generational trauma as well as the traumas we experienced in adulthood so that we can empower and liberate ourselves.

It all comes back to childhood and the survival mechanisms we learned to make ourselves feel safe in unsafe environments or stressful conditions, even in situations where our parents genuinely did the best they could. This includes the unresolved ancestral trauma that was passed down generationally through repetitive patterns, dynamics, habits, and subconscious belief programs.

Reflecting back to 2020, how have you responded since then?

Do you see any similar patterns to how you learned to respond to your childhood and ancestral trauma? How did that make you feel safe?

How has your life changed since 2020? The answer to this question will tell you how you're responding to the current evolutionary pressure. This will help you to gain insights that will help you to move through these ongoing liminal spaces.

The awesome thing is that you can always make new choices!

So, if you don't like the choices you made in the past—and that can include this morning or up until right now—you can start making different choices. The liminality of our current predicament is a gift, offering us the opportunity to make shifts toward what we want to create in our lives.

What we've done in the past led us to now, but that's not what is going to move us forward. If we keep doing the same thing, that will only lead to more repetition of what we don't want. This burden of the unresolved past becomes exponentially larger for individuals and society as long as we don't deal with it in constructive ways.

The present calling to grow up is about recognizing how we are participating in the chaos of the world through our personal lives, so that we can expand our awareness and make new choices. It's not our fault what's happening; but it is our responsibility to do something about it so that we can create the life we want to live and the kind of world we want to pass on to future generations.

Identifying the underlying sabotage programs

Self-sabotage programs are the remnants of childhood trauma and ancestral patterns that were passed down through the family lineage. Clearing subconscious programs and replacing them with upgraded ones that serve our growth and evolution is a *big* part of transforming the maladaptive behaviors that we all have.

But first, it's important to get mobilized out of the collapsed, checked out, or functional freeze state. As we explored in the last chapter on self-worth, we usually need a reason—a why—to get back up and return to living.

It's much easier to do the challenging inner work when you have energy and a healthy physical body, or at the very least, a solid system of self-care practices supporting you as you're working on building these.

To thrive in life, we also need healthy social connections. If you want to be able to deeply connect in healthy ways with people, the key is to identify your defensive responses. These are the primal mechanisms that are triggered when we feel threatened because something in the current environment (physical, social, mental, technological, or spiritual) reminds our nervous system of the unresolved past.

It's very often caused by our own thinking, the stories we tell ourselves in our inner dialogue, and how we *perceive* the events. Again, this isn't blame, shame, or judgment. We can observe with compassion and curiosity so that we can recognize how these primal states become self-sabotaging to our growth, relationships, and evolution.

It's important to identify the belief programs that are causing you to repeat the same old cycles and keep you stuck. You'll hear these in your self-talk when you're paying attention. Your triggers come from these subconscious programs, which were automatically installed due to stressful life events and the story we made up about what it means about us. Some of them were passed down ancestrally, as well. You may notice that you have programs and fears that come from what your ancestors experienced generations ago without you having had that experience.

These are some common subconscious programs:

"It's dangerous to speak the truth."

"I have to do everything on my own."

"My needs don't matter."

"I don't have the right to exist."

"It's not safe to be in my body."

"It's all my fault."

"Something is wrong with me."

"I'm unworthy."

"I'm unlovable."

"Nobody cares about me."

"I'm alone in the world."

You'll hear these kinds of thoughts in your inner dialogue if you're paying attention. They are usually triggered through interpersonal relationships and other social experiences. If you listen to your ruminating thoughts, you'll hear the story you're telling yourself about what's happening or happened.

These programs are like a narrative that you made up about yourself based on what happened to you, usually in childhood. Children feel like what's happening in their environment is their fault. In our early years, we often internalize the stresses of our parents and families. We make decisions that we aren't usually aware of, which help us to survive and feel safe, yet they sabotage our health and wellbeing later as they continue to play out in our relationships and how we respond to life.

Of course, these same programs will often keep getting reinforced in adulthood because they're like signals that your subconscious projects and others pick up on, even if they aren't consciously aware.

For example, if you have poor boundaries because no one ever taught you that you're allowed to have boundaries, that you're allowed to say no without punishment, then you'll probably encounter quite a few people who have no respect for your boundaries, who try to crush your dignity and autonomy, because this is a perfect vibrational match.

As the "mind architect" Peter Crone says so eloquently, "Life will present you with people and circumstances to reveal where you're not free."

This isn't a punishment and it's not your fault. It's part of the growth and evolutionary process. When you are triggered, the trigger is calling your attention to your programing, to all the places where you aren't free to make choices without the distortion of past stories. All of this can be upgraded so you can enjoy more ease, grace, expansion and, abundance in life.

It will be to your greatest benefit to recognize and unpack the negative and limiting programs when they come up through triggering experiences. You'll discover the underlying patterns if you allow yourself the self-honesty and humility necessary to see the things you don't want to see in yourself. It's worth it and you're worth it!

Once you identify a pattern, you can journal about where that came from, who taught you that, how it got reinforced in your life through more experiences, as well as the symptoms of that program manifesting in your life now.

With reverse engineering you can notice how the program triggers an emotional and behavioral response. Remind yourself that this self-reflection process isn't about self-blame or self-judgment. Steer yourself out of the old self-pity, shame, or harshness toward yourself, and redirect yourself toward curiosity and compassion.

Then you can create a new program to replace the old one. When you catch yourself having those negative thoughts again, immediately cancel or delete the thought, and replace it with your new program leading you toward growth. It's helpful to gather evidence of how the old program is a lie. Sometimes these shifts are easy to make, sometimes they are not.

When the negative program persists, that's a sign to do a deeper digging process into its origins. That will help you to gain more insights by discovering how it's serving you to keep that program running.

At first you might think, but it's *not* serving me! You're correct that *it just ain't working anymore* because it's subtracting more than adding to your life. Yet it is serving you in a distorted way. The subconscious is trying to solve problems and keep us safe, though there's usually a defensive undercurrent trying to fix things in ways that lead us away from what we really want.

What's the benefit of the negative program?

What do you get out of it?

Does it make you feel safe to self-isolate so that you don't get hurt?

Does anger motivate you to be successful and prove others wrong?

Does feeling unworthy make you dim your light, so that you don't feel like a tall poppy that will get cut down?

Does feeling defective give you a reason not to try, so that you can avoid the fear of failure?

These are just some common stances I've observed in myself and others over the years. In the ThetaHealing® technique classes, created by Vianna Stibal, I learned that we need to identify the benefit of the program in order to reprogram it, otherwise it will keep coming back. That's why the emphasis on *how is it serving you* is so helpful.

There are many different ways of doing subconscious digging and reprogramming. My favorite modality is the ThetaHealing technique. The process is so efficient for restoring lightness and inner freedom, layer by layer. You're also doing the work with the Creator, reminding you that you're never alone and you don't need to exhaust yourself by *efforting* so much with your willpower or self-reliance. When we create the space for spirit to enter, it's so much easier to transform our lives.

I also love David Bayer's work about powerful vs. primal states, which he teaches in his podcast, his book *A Changed Mind*, his coaching programs, and at his Powerful Living Experience events.

Becoming a responsible adult

Before we can do the deeper restorative work of integrating the inner child, we first need to get the adult in the driver's seat.

Many of us grew up with childhood trauma that set us up to come of age as dysfunctional adults. We also live in a socially engineered world where we are infantilized and conditioned to react like children who are dependent on Big Daddy government.

Sometimes we jump straight into marriage and kids without doing the inner work, and then the burden is passed on and the cycle continues. Other times we know we aren't ready for parenthood, but we get into quite a few painful and re-traumatizing experiences in adulthood that add to the burden that we are already carrying. We might start to believe something is wrong with us because we rack up more experiences that can be perceived through that lens, seemingly providing more evidence of that program, which is a lie.

I've heard some people say that the problem with our world is that we humans are too emotional. I disagree. Emotion is part of the richness of the human experience, and it's possible to experience emotions in a responsible, exquisite, and beneficial way. The challenge is when we feel threatened and get triggered unconsciously, then react like toddlers throwing temper tantrums, or like destructive, aggressive adolescents.

Psychologist Terry Real, who was inspired by his mentor Pia Mellody, describes his framework of the *functional adult*, *wounded child*, and *adaptive child*. Real's work focuses on the adolescent—the adaptive child, to help people to change the behaviors that are currently sabotaging their relationships.

My perspective of these states of human awareness is similar, but different based on the work I've done with myself and other people. When it comes to childhood trauma, I find it's very important to work with the young version of the inner child as well as the baby in the womb. This is where I've found the deeper roots of the repetitive and self-sabotaging behaviors and programs.

Our current global and personal crises are indicative of a species living in captivity caused by unresolved trauma, then reacting like wounded children and angry adolescents. We are caught in this distorted trauma dance in our relationship with ourselves, our interpersonal relationships and in world relations.

The escalation of these crises is an invitation to grow into healthy, functional adults who can integrate the childlike parts of themselves that didn't get their needs met once upon a time, then evolving into our higher self. When we learn to meet our own needs instead of expecting others to do that for us or projecting our pain and shadow on others, we can self-actualize and form healthy, functional relationships where we are free and able to contribute and amplify one another and our shared experience in positive ways.

Healthy, functional adults can feel, process, and express emotions in responsible and respectful ways. Numbing emotions is not a sign of health or maturity but an avoidance of our trauma and humanity.

The threshold into functional adulthood is self-responsibility. This happens when a person finally sees the insanity of doing the same thing and expecting different results. That victimhood- and prison-shattering realization opens the door to the new possibilities that come with taking responsibility for our choices and life.

This is the threshold of empowerment. It starts with a new decision and commitment to taking 100 percent responsibility for our life and choices. It doesn't mean we are perfect, and it doesn't mean we have it all figured out—it means we can take responsibility for ourselves, even when we mess up, and that we believe in our ability to figure things out.

A responsible adult is capable of managing life responsibilities and personal needs with ease and grace. In relationships, a responsible adult can communicate directly and explicitly, collaborating well with others.

A responsible adult has healthy boundaries and respects the boundaries of others. A healthy, functional adult is assertive, neither aggressive nor passive. A responsible adult has a sense of duty and compassion yet is willing to draw the line when something isn't okay. A responsible adult has discernment and doesn't trust everyone, because not everyone is trustworthy.

A responsible adult has self-worth and self-esteem. A responsible adult is empowered, self-disciplined, exploratory, and seeks access to higher consciousness and an intimate connection with God, the Creator of All That Is, Spirit, Source, Infinite Intelligence, or whatever you call your higher power.

A responsible adult knows right from wrong, has empathy and knowledge, and is capable of self-regulation. A responsible adult evaluates the consequences of actions and responds, instead of reacting, to people and life.

Keep in mind that your adult self will continue maturing and growing along the way during your evolutionary journey and you don't have to have it all figured out or do it perfectly. A responsible adult can admit to mistakes while having the self-compassion to recognize that mistakes are just choices and you can always learn from the past and make new choices.

Once you have created solid ground through the empowerment of self-responsibility, then you can do the inner child work because your adult self is capable of being the stable, compassionate witness with the inner resources to rescue and care for the unintegrated child parts.

In which areas of your life do you feel like a responsible and functional adult?

Are there any areas of your life where you wish others would rescue you from your circumstances or feelings?

Who is responsible for your life circumstances and your happiness?

When you feel threatened, who do you become?

RESPONSIBLE ADULT

Responsible / Empowered
Safe & Social
Attuned & Interdependent
Functional & Resourced
Resilient
Exploratory
Encouraging
Mature & Self-Regulated
Nuanced
Discernment and Boundaries
Access to Higher Consciousness
Connected / Healthy Co-Regulation

Needs: Responsibility and Autonomy

Integrating the inner child

Rescuing and integrating your inner child is another important part of growing up after childhood trauma.

This process involves integrating the exiled parts of your soul that checked out when things were too painful or scary. These are the parts of you that are sabotaging your life and causing you to look for an external savior. There are usually quite a few of these soul fragments, especially with severe childhood trauma. This restorative work is ongoing, layer by layer.

The young versions of the inner child are the ones who need a sense of safety. They are stuck, frozen in time with unmet needs that no one was able or willing to recognize. It's not your fault what happened, yet it is your responsibility now as an adult to connect with these parts of yourself, to validate their feelings and to recognize their unmet needs so you can reassure them (yourself) and give them (yourself) the love they (you) needed.

When I do this work with responsible adults, I ask them to connect with the sensations and feelings emerging from their body through a guided meditation for embodiment. The sensations and feelings connect to earlier memories where those energetic imprints took place. It's often surprising and not what people were expecting to see, but these were pivotal life moments that set off a chain reaction of events, decisions, patterns, and beliefs that a person carries through life.

Responsible adults can empathize with what their inner child was feeling and recognize the unmet needs. Then, from an observer perspective, they can visualize being the adult they didn't have in that moment, stepping into the scene to rescue the child. Sometimes they simply need a hug and reassurance that they're loved. In severe cases of trauma, such as abuse, the adult observer will want to remove the child from that scene and take her somewhere she wants to go where she feels safe, like a park, to grandma's house, or to get ice cream.

It may take some time to earn the child's trust. This is especially true when we don't trust ourselves due to the ways we have abandoned, rejected, or betrayed ourselves as a result of our programming.

Sometimes trust happens very quickly, as soon as the adult is able to attune with, recognize, and meet the unmet needs of the child. Then the adult creates a new frame of the past where the child now feels loved, cherished, worthy, seen, heard, and held.

The subconscious can't tell the difference between what you're vividly imagining and what's really happening, so this process creates a new meaning of the past. We can't change what happened, but we do have the power to shift what it means, which changes who we are, how we perceive life, and how we live. As we upgrade the meaning of the past, we open new possibilities for the future.

You'll know you're having a deep, restorative connection with your inner child when the tears start. That's usually when we recognize how vulnerable the child was, how alone the child felt, and how we've let our inner child down unintentionally, simply because we continued our pattern into adulthood without realizing it.

After the recognition and re-establishment of attunement, trust, and love, the adult can bring the little child back into his heart, offering the child a forever home where his needs will be seen, heard, and met. The adult can promise to take care of the child so the child can be free to be childlike again. It's also helpful for the adult to ask the child to *gently* get his attention when he needs it. This process of self-awareness begins to interrupt the old automatic self-sabotage patterns and create a new relationship with oneself.

WOUNDED INNER CHILD

Fawn / Compliance
Freeze / Dissociation / Fantasy
Collapse / Shutdown
Immobilization
Numbness
Hopelessness / Despair
Invisible / Vulnerable
Complaining / Demanding
Insecure / Dependent
Tantrums
All-or-Nothing Thinking
Alone / Lost / Disconnected

Needs: Safety and Reassurance

The self-sabotaging adolescent versions of the inner child are the rebellious, destructive ones who want a sense of control, though deep down they also want to be recognized and know that they matter. These are the protective parts that are sabotaging your life and relationships by wanting to be right and win at any cost.

We usually don't realize how the desire to be right becomes a self-fulfilling prophecy where we continually prove that we are right, in all the ways that we don't actually want.

These needs can be severely distorted. You might discover that your adolescent parts are trying to prove that they're right that no one cares about you, and in the process you're sabotaging your relationships by fighting and pushing everyone away. Likewise, when the adolescent has experienced injustice, he usually continues to gravitate toward more experiences of injustice, proving that he's right that life sucks and that people take advantage of him.

Perfectionism and rigid, black-and-white, thinking comes from the inner adolescent. Most of our addictions also come from the adolescent parts. Addictions mask and numb the pain. These give us a sense of control and agency over our lives, but at a tremendous cost.

Self-hatred usually comes from the adolescent parts who learned that it was easier to hate themselves than admit they hate someone (usually parents and peers) who hurt them—because it wasn't safe at the time to recognize how they were being abused or otherwise hurt.

Working with the inner adolescent is a little different. You can negotiate with these parts. You'll be able to have more verbal interactions with them. They'll want to understand things and you'll be able to explain more to them if you're not so triggered that you're trying to destroy everything.

First, you'll want to meet the inner adolescent parts where they are. Listen to them, show interest in them, and find out what they really want, not just what they *think* they want (which is usually based on distortion) or what *you* think they should do (which will only trigger the defense mechanisms). Encourage their strengths and gifts as well as their growth process. Then teach them to get what they want in a healthy new way. It's very helpful to practice visualization when you're connecting with the adolescent parts as well.

You can thank the inner adolescent parts for figuring out how to survive when things were very challenging. You can validate how they helped you to survive by engaging in those specific (defensive) behaviors. Also tell them what it's costing you to keep repeating those patterns in your life and relationships. Then let them know that you've got this now, that you can handle the adult responsibilities, and be the adult so they don't have to. Over time, you'll earn their trust as you show them that they can count on you to lead the way, so they can relax, have more fun, and individuate in healthy ways.

SELF-SABOTEUR ADOLESCENT

Defensive & Walled Off
Fight and Flight
Mobilization
Self-Protective
Destructive & Rebellious
Self-Righteous
Wants to Win at Any Cost
Perfectionism & Self-Hatred
Avoidance / Escaping
Hyper-Independence
Rigid Thinking
Misunderstood / Angry / Disconnected

Needs: Control and Recognition

Integrating your inner child at various ages and key moments is a process that you'll be able to deepen as you go. It's like developing a relationship over time. You'll become more adept at noticing when those younger parts of yourself are asking for your attention before they act out and make a mess of things.

When you miss the cue, you'll soon see how they're driving your life. The child parts get triggered and defensive, not the adult. When you self-regulate, you're being the adult that co-regulates with your inner child in the way that your caretakers didn't when you were a kid.

The adult should be the one driving the car. When you recognize that's not the case, get yourself back in the driver's seat ASAP by returning to the empowerment of self-responsibility. Then work with the inner child parts so that they can feel safe, reassured, recognized, and trust you to have their back. This inner work can be challenging, so it can be helpful to have a guide to walk you through the process.

The more integrated we are, the less we live stuck in our childlike parts and the primal brain, which means more access to higher states of consciousness. When we are operating from our inner adult, we are empowered, whole, and resourced.

Expanding into your higher self

The more conditioning and programming that we release and reprogram, the more wholeness we restore to our soul, and the more effortlessly we can upshift into our inner sage or higher self.

What's wild is that the higher self is wise, yet has a childlike freedom and expansion. It has elements of the child before the trauma programming and conditioning happened, when the child felt limitless and boundless. Ideally, children are born knowing their inherent worth and feeling free to express themselves. It is our life experiences that teach us otherwise.

However, for many of us, the distortions started with energetic imprints of a hostile environment in utero. Part of the inner child integration work involves clearing those imprints from our experiences in the womb. The moment we are conceived, when the two cells merge into one, there's an instant energetic download—something like a zip file—of all the genetic information from the mother and father's lineage.

A healthy, loved, and supported child, much like the inner sage, is spontaneous and playful, has natural discernment and has access to limitless imagination. *From the mouths of babes* come bold, extraordinary insights that some adults dare not speak out loud.

The inner sage is awakened, neutral, wise, self-actualized, and present. This is the part of us that uplifts and inspires others, that lives in communion with the Creator of All That Is. It's the part of us that lives in higher consciousness, that can observe from the perspective of non-duality and duality at the same time.

While it's necessary to be a responsible adult to function well in this world, cultivating the inner sage isn't required for survival. This is the part of us that wants to *thrive*. Thriving is optional in life. This is the part of us that wants to discover and activate our divine purpose and mission. It's the aspect of self that feels a calling to contribute to humanity in some way. While the adult self has access to states of higher consciousness, the inner sage lives in these states.

If you feel a calling to be of service to others based on your unique talents, gifts, and interests, that's coming from your higher self. You might feel a bit alone on that path for a while if you realize that you're surrounded by people who are more in a child, adolescent, or adult state.

While the adult likes rules, the inner sage may feel confined by the rules because this part of us is more interested in what is morally right—not in rigidity, dogma, or mental constructs. It's more about accessing the virtue of prudence, the situational conscience that John Bradshaw wrote about.

The higher self is focused on cultivating virtues such as wisdom, prudence, compassion, and expansion. This part of us wants to bring out the best in other people who are receptive. When we are in a sage state, we don't want to hang out with people who aren't receptive, uplifting, or mutually inspiring. In fact, the more we embody the inner sage, the smaller and more refined our inner circle might become.

INNER SAGE / HIGHER SELF

Awakened & Grounded
Self-Assured
Kind / Loving / Forgiving
Neutral
Wise
Growth-Focused
Present & Aware
Cultivating Inner Peace
Uplifts & Inspires Others
Deep Connection with All That Is
Living in Higher States of Consciousness

Needs: Aligned Relationships and Purpose

It's not that one part of ourselves is better than another, or that we should try to be in a sage state all the time, bypassing our inner work. It's also not blame or judgment to recognize when we are triggered in another state. That's part of having a human experience. We will feel whole and thriving when we are growing, strengthening, and integrating *all* aspects of who we are—inner child, inner adolescent, responsible adult, and inner sage.

What percentage of your day do you spend in a wounded child state? In a self-saboteur adolescent state? In a responsible adult state? In a higher self state?

What kind of effect do the people in your life have on you? Are they more like children, adolescents, adults, or sages?

Self-care is the foundation of growth

Much of what's happening in our personal lives and the world is out of our control. That can feel disempowering and trigger our maladaptive defense mechanisms.

If we don't have a solid system of self-care to use as a foundation of support through the stress, next comes the self-destruction and self-sabotage from unintegrated soul parts.

Self-care isn't about spa time and pampering, though there's nothing wrong with that. Self-care is about inner nourishing practices that build self-love over time and provide a solid foundation to guide us through challenging times.

This includes things like regular exercise; good nutrition; quality sleep; meditation; journaling; contemplation; setting boundaries; rebuilding self-worth, self-esteem, and self-trust; and taking inventory of our social connections and inner circle. Most important, we must do the inner work of taking responsibility for ourselves and our choices, recognizing our maladaptive defense mechanisms, integrating the inner child and growing into healthy adults who can access and activate our higher self's sense of purpose and mission.

What is your self-care system and where does it live on your calendar?

How well are you administering your internal and external resources?

Is your environment (physical, mental, emotional, spiritual, social, technological) designed intentionally to support your self-care system or are you relying on willpower to maintain it?

How is your current relationship with your body?

Don't waste time and energy beating yourself up for not doing it sooner. That's not productive and only adds to the shame. *Speaking from experience.* Redirect those resources to doing it now so that you can build greater resilience and grow with a solid foundation to support you. It won't be long before you'll be really glad you did.

From post-trauma to post-traumatic growth

Post-traumatic growth is about transforming the pain of the past by making new choices, doing the inner work, and updating the self-concept after trauma. It's about awakening, self-discovery, and evolution. Along the way, we clarify our values and strengthen our integrity, creating a new sense of identity, meaning, and purpose. The past no longer has the same effect on our body, behavior, or identity.

But that's not the choice that most people are making right now. Most are stuck under layers of denial, defensiveness, and cognitive dissonance. Even among those who are awake and aware of what's been happening, most are still focused externally on what *they* are doing to us. I have compassion for that because I was there, too. It's just that getting stuck there is *really* unproductive.

It's challenging to heal on a battlefield. However, I don't recommend we wait to do our inner growth work until everything is fine in the world. That day may or may not come. We can minimize our exposure as much as possible to the toxic and harmful elements as our world is going through massive changes, while doing the inner work. This is our challenge, and this is our evolutionary calling.

I delayed my next stage of growth when things started in 2020, and I had to work extra hard to overcome that self-sabotage setback. The further down that path we go, the longer it takes to find our way back. But the amazing thing is that no matter how far down the wrong path we've gone, we can always make the decision to return to center and make new choices.

The first step toward growth is the perspective shift. Admittedly, I was stuck in a negative paradigm for the first few years of the 2020s. But now I see things differently.

As the saying goes, it's happening *for* you, not to you. This is one of the most important perspective shifts to get re-oriented from powerlessness to power.

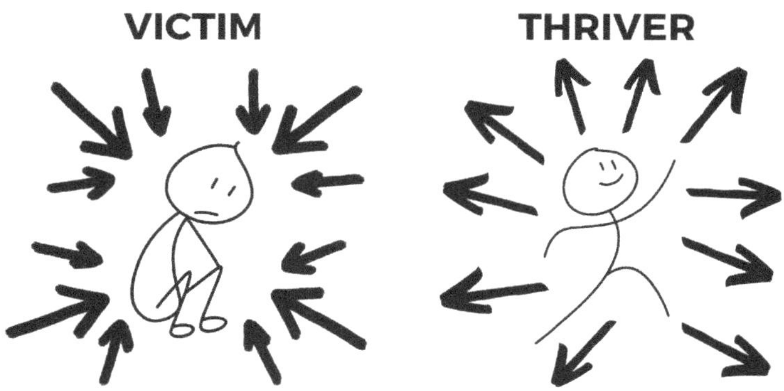

When something is happening *to* us, we are in a victim state of consciousness. When it's happening *for* us, we are in an empowered state of consciousness. The same thing is happening in both circumstances. The only difference is the perspective.

Perspective is a choice. It's one of the most vital choices we can make during these times if we want to heal, grow, live a more joyful life, and leave a better legacy for future generations.

Last year, I took a road trip off the beaten path through the Northwest of the United States. Many fires burned down the forests up there, some more recent than others. It was harsh to see the black, naked trees and barren land, while smelling the smoke for hundreds of miles and knowing that the destruction was ongoing.

But there was also something amazing happening.

Alongside the mountain highways lined with black ash, rows and rows of golden flowers emerged. Glancing further out into the forest, I could see little signs of new life being created and emerging from the destruction.

Nature knows how to heal itself.

Our bodies have a similar homeostasis principle. However, the difference with humans is that we also have consciousness, which either amplifies or interrupts the self-healing mechanism. *It depends on how we use our power.*

When we have layers of frozen trauma in the subconscious and body, the homeostatic self-healing mechanism is hindered. For the most part, we have forgotten how to use our consciousness for self-healing and growth.

In fact, we are continually bombarded with negative messaging, poisonous chemicals, and electromagnetic frequencies that suppress our ability to heal ourselves and thrive. Make no mistake, that is all by design. But it's not happening to us because we deserve it—it's happening *for* us to invite us to grow and evolve, to step into our power and liberate ourselves from the darkness of captivity.

Shifting into power

Powerlessness is where we can get stuck without realizing it because it feels empowering to recognize the abuse. That's not real power though. It's simply an external awareness, which is helpful for setting boundaries to protect yourself, yet not healing.

After 2020, I learned how strong the primal brain programmed by trauma is, and how my subconscious was ruining my life. I realized I had deeper layers of healing to do so I could stop that cycle and regain conscious control over my choices. I needed to completely rebuild my self-worth from the inside.

It blew my mind how quickly we can forget what matters most when things get really stressful. That's usually because of the layers of unhealed trauma from childhood and the ancestral DNA memory hijacking the brain and nervous system in an attempt to survive.

I learned that lesson the hard way, as many of us often do. I went back into victimhood, focusing externally on what the perpetrators were doing and wishing someone was coming to save us from the evil forces oppressing society and individuals. I had a rescue fantasy that brave, strong men would stand up and protect the rest of us from the abusers. But much like in my family system, that didn't happen. No one is coming to save us. Yet amazing synchronicities and opportunities can show up when we are in a faith-centered state instead of a fear-centered state. That's why this work starts internally.

After clearing more layers of unresolved trauma through embodiment, self-regulation, reprogramming my subconscious beliefs, and integrating my inner child, I realized I don't want to learn the hard way anymore. That was based on the old trauma programming. It was just a program that I believed was life. So, I unsubscribed and made the decision to learn through ease, grace, and inspiration.

As crazy as that time was, there was also something amazing happening.

It was an opportunity to recognize how I was still sabotaging myself, and the parts of me that needed healing, growth, and strengthening so that I could restore wholeness and return to my true self. But let me tell you, that was not easy!

I got stuck for a while and lost my way. It was a struggle, and even in the moment, I knew I wasn't making the most of it. I knew I was forgetting so many tools and skills that I'd learned over the prior two decades of personal development and spiritual growth work. I knew I was going back into victim consciousness. But even still, I couldn't help myself from drifting into it!

The wiser part of me—my higher self—wasn't easily accessible while I was in a primal state. I would only catch glimpses of awareness that peaked through the clouds. My ego and survival self were driving, and those parts of me were trying to fix the situation in *all* the wrong ways.

Thankfully, I heard the inner calling and was motivated to make bigger bets on myself, personally and professionally, so that I could use the challenges as an opportunity to grow and guide others through this challenging terrain that we are all facing in our own unique ways.

Recently I heard someone suggest looking back in the photos on your phone to a certain time of your life and noticing how different you are now.

I chose 2020. Looking at those photos inspired a deeper dive into my reflections on that time, which led to integrating more insights and recognizing how much I've grown.

Then I asked myself, "How did it serve me?"

Everything that happens, and everything we choose, serves us in some way. It's a matter of perspective.

If I could be a guardian angel visiting my 2020 self, I would whisper that question in her ear.

How is it serving you?

CHAPTER 16

NAVIGATING THE LIMINAL SPACES

The Only Way Out Is Through

We are living in wild times on planet Earth. Fresh on the heels of the COVID tyranny and abuse, we are rapidly entering another massive paradigm shift unlike anything our ancestors experienced.

The advancements in technology and AI in the coming years are going to change our lives in ways that we can't even imagine yet because it will be an entirely new experience. This is also going to be the next frontier of captivity. We'd be wise to recognize both the advantages and perils that come with new technology so that we can approach the changes with wisdom and discernment.

In Chapter 9, we explored the liminality of these times, this strange unsettling state in which we find ourselves right now after the existentially shattering experiences of the early 2020s. It's only going to get weirder in the years to come.

In the middle of this convergence point in human history, the unresolved past of our ancestry is triggered and rising to the surface. We are either going to upload the darkness of the past into the new quantum computing mainframe, or create a new future based on how we actually want to live.

Humans have been living in a state of captivity for a long time, escalating with each added historical trauma that goes on unmetabolized from one generation to the next. The choice to emerge and evolve from this story is ours. It's the calling of a lifetime as we are on the bridge between two worlds.

All of us are under tremendous evolutionary pressure in the 2020s. This is a cosmic invitation that will require facing your deepest fear—whatever holds the greatest power over your life—so that you can unlock your power and liberate yourself. If you reflect with honesty, you've probably already seen these themes surfacing.

If we want to survive and thrive through the present and ongoing challenges, we will need to learn how to navigate the liminal spaces in the world as well as in our hearts and minds.

Ladies and gentlemen, please fasten your seatbelts as we are entering an area of turbulence.

It's going to be a bumpy ride. While that's unsettling and potentially dangerous, the human spirit is built for this journey. I believe those of us who are alive right now chose this mission before incarnating. There are many souls wishing they could have a turn to come here now to participate in these historical times.

Yet right now most of us are sleepwalking through the dark night, plugged into devices and tuned out of deep connection with one another, with ourselves, with our Creator, as well as what's happening in the world.

Ignoring, suppressing, avoiding, or masking by trying to go on like nothing is happening will not lead us to healing, growth, and evolution. We are going to need to face it. It's only going to get louder until we do.

The only way out is through.

But what does that really mean?

Leaning in

Many people feel like nothing makes sense anymore. Indeed, it feels like we are living in surreal times.

Like abuse survivors waking up to the truth about the abuse and starting to realize the impact of the trauma on their entire life, or a person who lost a dear loved one, or a society experiencing massive turmoil, a sense of surrealism sets in as we wonder what's next. It's deeply disruptive and uncomfortable.

As individuals, and as a collective, we are currently walking through the liminal spaces—the transitional states and places between the old and the new, the familiar and the unknown—where we are being forced out of our comfort zones.

There's also an unsettling liminal state after giving up our escapist behaviors and unhealthy habits. When you're no longer the person who drinks too much, overeats, seeks external validation, or participates in toxic relationships in order to avoid the feelings of loneliness and pain, you'll be forced to face the things you didn't want to see about yourself, now without the distractions. This can be unnerving and may cause people to return to old habits or to find new ways of doing the same thing.

The mirror of self-honesty is not always easy to look into. It's important to understand that *the person bruised by trauma is not the real you.* The ugliness you see after giving up the distractions is just your programming and emotional residue. That's how the trauma shaped you. Underneath *all* of that is the real you.

As you give up unhealthy choices and habits, you enter the liminal space between the old you and the new you. It's worth doing the inner work of the healing journey to discover your true self and update your identity into the person you're becoming.

You can create the life that you want to live, and this is one of the greatest gifts of evolutionary pressure during these disruptive and unsettling times. Most of us were not living consciously before 2020, even when we thought we were awakened. We are now being challenged to dig deeper and expand beyond our limitations.

Learning to navigate the liminal spaces is key for thriving in this decade of transformation. We are moving through a dimensional portal of limitless potential. It's inviting us to do a deep questioning of identity, meaning and purpose, freedom and responsibility, life and death, as well as our worldview.

The liminal spaces can feel incredibly uncertain, bringing up much fear. That can trick you into thinking that you're powerless to do anything to positively affect your life, or that you have to control everything in order to feel safe and protected. Remember that your choices are where you'll find your power. One of the most essential choices we can make daily is whether to align with fear or with faith.

No matter what is going on around you, you can choose to cultivate a sense of true empowerment by *owning the power of your choices*. You can choose to create new meaning in the face of anxiety and uncertainty. You can choose to believe that everything is going to work out as you take aligned action steps toward your goals and dreams, trusting that life is going to meet you where you are.

You can choose to confront the negative and dark forces within yourself so that you can transmute them into light. The external darkness loses its power over you as you reclaim your territory, inner resources, and sovereignty—most significantly by aligning your inner authority with your faith in the Creator of All That Is. We don't have to fight the darkness. It loses power and goes away as we shift from fear to faith through our daily choices.

Making new existential choices starts in our thoughts, decisions, actions, investment of time and energy, and how we connect through relationships. Your day is the sum of your awareness, perspective, decisions, actions, and connections. In other words, it's about how you respond to yourself, others, and life, and how you choose to show up in each moment.

Leaning in and rising to the challenge with faith instead of giving up is the only way to get through these times without suffering. As many of the great sages have said, pain is inevitable, but suffering is optional. It has a lot to do with the way we frame our experiences through our perspective.

If we try to hold on to the old, replay the past, or feed our fears, that will lead to depression and anxiety, to a lot of really dark, frustrating, and scary places. We can't go back to how things were before 2020. But that doesn't have to be a bad thing. What's happening could become the best thing that's ever happened because it's forcing us to become more aware and to evolve.

To move through these challenges with greater ease and grace, we'll need to learn to become professionals at navigating liminal spaces.

Becoming a PRO at navigating liminal spaces

You can turn to this acronym any time you feel stuck or when things feel overwhelming, scary, and challenging.

1. Shift your PERSPECTIVE to shift your state.

Notice when you're in states of fear, defensiveness, victim consciousness, negative and primal thinking, or catastrophizing. Recognize when you're giving energy to a past-oriented focus, rumination, and shame-based, fear-centered, or critical thoughts, and when you are afraid to set boundaries or speak up because of how others will react.

Rewrite the story you're telling yourself with curiosity and compassion. Notice how it's happening *for* you, not to you. Check in to see where your perspective is coming from: the inner child (the wounded little one or the self-sabotaging adolescent), the responsible adult, or the higher self. Redefine yourself in the story with empowerment and self-worth. Revisit your core personal values and remind yourself of what matters to you most. Give yourself permission to say no more often. Remind yourself that you don't have to own other people's feelings, thoughts, opinions, pain, and projections. Keep redirecting yourself from fear to faith to create the space for divine grace to enter.

Perspective Shift: What are you most grateful for right now?

2. Change your ROUTINE to change your results.

Notice where your time goes daily. Identify your unhealthy habits, distractions, and coping mechanisms. Pay attention to how you show up in your life—at your job or business, in your relationships (intimate partnerships, friendships, family), and with your community. Do an audit of your self-care practices and whether you have what Napoleon Hill calls "definiteness of purpose" or if you're drifting in life.

Administer your energy and time with clarity, intention, and meaning. Start with your calendar. You can create color-coded chunks of time for self-care and health habits, growth and learning, work and wealth-building, purpose, creativity and play, organization and planning, contemplation, meditation, *presencing*, prayer, authentic relationships, and family.

Check in to see if what really matters to you is given space on your calendar. Make more space to allow room for new consciousness and inspiration. Notice where you're overcommitted or committed to things you don't want to be doing. Recognize how much time you spend on social media and doing other things online. Your devices are probably tracking these stats for you. Then make adjustments to get new results. Especially pay attention to what you do with your idle time because that's when the darkness can creep in unnoticed.

Routine Shift: How do you fill the existential void?

3. OBSERVE yourself through mindfulness.

Notice where you have a lack of awareness about yourself and your life. Sometimes you don't see it, but other people might point it out to you. That could be good feedback.

Observe your environment (physical, social, emotional, mental, spiritual, and technological) to notice the effects it has on you. Gauge your level of engagement and enthusiasm in your projects and purpose. Call yourself out and get back to purpose when you realize that you're drifting through distractions.

Meditation and contemplation can be helpful for the practice of observation and the building of mindfulness. You can use your breath as a tool. Schedule *unplugged time* on your calendar when you turn off the phone, email, and other distractions to be present with yourself and sit in solitude. Put your phone in another room—otherwise, you'll find that you're compulsively reaching for it. You can do the same when you're connecting with your loved ones. Put the phone away and you'll see how different your experience is.

It's helpful to write about your insights and do regular journaling practices to continually evaluate what you're accomplishing, how you're growing, and what you're letting go of that no longer serves you or leads you back to the past. Reflect and write about what you really want to create in your life and what's stopping you from having that now.

Observe how you're approaching yourself and others. Can you lead with more honesty and directness? This doesn't mean being a jerk. It means having direct, explicit communication with yourself and others instead of avoiding important topics or conflicts, or slipping into ambiguity and misunderstanding. Have clarifying conversations instead of omitting information you're afraid to say or ask about because of how you think the other person will react. Listen to what others are saying and ask more questions. This is a way of bringing more mindfulness and authenticity into your relationships.

Some conversations are simply not necessary at all. When you're radically honest with yourself, you might realize that it would be a waste of your time to try to talk openly and directly with a person who is evasive and unwilling to accept personal responsibility for his or her actions. Those kinds of conversations usually lead to more frustration, pain, exhaustion, and crazymaking.

Ask yourself: What were the top three best choices you have made since 2020? Journal about your responses so you can gain more awareness and insights. Give yourself validation for how you chose and choose to grow during the challenging times.

Was there anything that you wish you did differently? Journal about this so you can explore the mistakes you made and reframe them with empowerment instead of victimhood and shame. This exercise can help you to visualize how you would do things differently next time. This is a valuable tool!

Observation Shift: What's the next best step that you can take toward greater authenticity now?

The new avant-garde for the terrain ahead

A few weeks before finishing the revisions of this book, I drove down to David Bayer's Powerful Living Experience in Austin, Texas. The whole event was fantastic, and his work is on the cutting edge of personal development. David and his wife, Carol, create a beautiful space for transformational work.

On the last day, they invited their somatic therapist, Aliah Whitmore, to facilitate a collective breath work practice. The stage was re-set, the lighting was dimmed, and meditation music was playing to set the tone. In a room of 800 people, we were each paired up with a partner to go through the process together. Aliah guided us with her voice and a gong to help us settle into the practice.

As we started the process, I felt tightness in my back behind my heart. I soon realized it was emotional pain surfacing. As we shifted from the parasympathetic to sympathetic breathing, the energy in the room began to get more intense. People started to emote and release. I suddenly felt so cold all the way into my bones. A sense of terror surfaced from my experience in the womb, a pattern I'd been working on deeper levels recently. My whole body began to shiver and tremble uncontrollably. Then it bent over toward a fetal position as I started sobbing.

My partner instantly held my hands tighter, squeezing gently to let me know he was there, and I wasn't alone. I was both in, and expanded beyond, my body, having my own experience while simultaneously hearing and feeling the echoes around the room as hundreds of people were crying, screaming, laughing, expressing in various ways, whatever was emerging for them. It felt like we were all having our own experience and at the same time, a collective shared *presencing*.

I had a fleeting thought that maybe I was a burden for my partner. As if he could read my mind, he squeezed my hands again. I finally understood what is meant by containment, the masculine art of creating and holding a container in which the feminine energy can feel safe and supported to self-express. He was like a living rock, solid yet also deeply attuned. It was the first time that that sensation of terror had surfaced without me feeling like I was floating alone in the abyss, untethered to anything or anyone else.

That womb imprint and feeling had haunted me all my life, though I didn't fully understand it until the month before the seminar when I had a huge breakthrough after a back crisis. I identified and cleared the program that surfaced from my sacrum and neck, then had a very positive experience with a chiropractor. She fixed my back with her healing touch and provided a new experience where it felt safe to ask for and receive support without the old distortions and fears. It laid the groundwork for the next level, which would happen during the breath work practice at the event. Feeling open, safe, supported, and connected, I received a new energetic imprint, overwriting the old one from the womb. I knew nothing would ever be the same.

After the practice concluded, we debriefed with our partners. When I opened my eyes, my partner looked at me and said, "That was otherworldly." He reached out and pulled me in for a bear hug. I thanked him for creating a safe container for me to have that experience. He replied, "Thank you for helping me *feel.* I hadn't felt anything in a long time."

Some people shared their experiences publicly. Many nodded as empathic witnesses. It was a powerful, intimate experience of liberation in divine synchronicity for everyone in that room—an example of *convulsive beauty*.

Over a decade ago, I used to facilitate eye-gazing seminars with small groups. Sometimes I would hear from people who tracked me down years later to tell me how powerful their experience was and how they never forgot it. I'd been feeling the calling to get back to this kind of work in person with people. The breath work experience was confirmation that it's time.

Healing arts and technologies like breath work and eye gazing come from ancient practices, yet they're avant-garde in our world where disconnection, materialism, programming, and the avoidance of our trauma are the norm. Artistic experiences like these can help us *presence* the emergent information and re-connect with our true essence where we remember who we are. It also brings us back together in deep, holistic connection to share a powerful ineffable experience of our humanity.

About a week after returning from the event, and just before moving away from Oklahoma, an early morning tornado touched down, bringing destruction just a few *blocks* from where I lived. My body's seasoned internal alarm woke me up about ten to fifteen minutes before the storm arrived.

When I heard the siren, I grabbed my dog and went to our safe room, an interior bathroom with no windows. I recognized the usual nervous system sympathetic activation, the intense chemicals and jittery sensations coursing through my body, as I opened an app on my phone to check the live emergency weather broadcast. Horrified, I realized the tornado was already on the ground and right there. Then, instantly, a calm came over me. My dog stopped panting and laid down with a sigh.

My nervous system had suddenly shifted into a state of peace. It wasn't a decision I made. I didn't use a coping mechanism or try to talk myself out of feeling fear. It just happened on its own. I knew I was either going to be safe from harm or it was the calm before death, in which case everything would be alright, too.

Normally it takes an hour after the threat has passed for the sympathetic response to turn off and shift out of the primal state. Then there are usually a few hours of hangover from the flooding of adrenaline. But none of that happened this time.

After the storm had passed, I went to make coffee and reflect. Something had shifted, but how? I realized it had to do with that breath work experience and the new energetic imprint I received, as well as the shift in my state after the event. With these updates to my nervous system, I can now access a new sense of inner safety.

Of course, I also believe there was an element of divine intervention. Tornadoes make a *lot* of noise. I don't know how else to explain how quiet and still everything was outside. The little rosemary pot on my porch that I have to pick up about once a week when the wind blows it around hadn't moved an inch.

The next day I drove about one minute down the road to the devastation where disaster crews were working. Massive trees were uprooted and laying on houses, fences were blown away, and roofs were blown off. I realized how very blessed I was. It also put things into new perspective for me. The fears had been trying to creep in as they do when we are making big life transitions. Now I realize how silly those fears are because I know what it feels like to have a deep sense of peace *one minute away from a tornado.*

Many people have been asking where a safe place is to go to during this global chaos. I don't think there is one, though certain areas may be more or less affected than others. Part of our evolutionary journey as individuals and humanity is to discover that there is no real safety and security in the external world. The only safe place is an inner experience of knowing that everything is going to be okay. Getting through the challenging times is also going to be a lot easier when we have aligned connections with others.

As much as I tried to mentally convince myself over the years that inner safety is the only real safety, the new experience of my nervous system during the tornado brought a visceral understanding. It was a confirmation of the shift that I received during the art of breathing together and all the events that led up to that moment. The safe social container during that experience upgraded the energetic imprint from inner terror to safety, which is now a code that I can carry forward with me and share with others.

I believe the avant-garde of the 2020s is a calling for deeper connection, healing, introspection, liberation, and systemic change *starting within the individual yet in the container of the collective.* This is essential for navigating the liminal spaces and transcending the repetition of cycles of destruction, from the micro to the macro, that inevitably happen when we look for an external savior or suppress and avoid the trauma, which then gets passed on to future generations.

Are you an avant-garde artist in your own unique way? I encourage you to take advantage of the liminality of these times, to tap into your authentic self as you integrate the past, so you can unleash new levels of your creativity to share with others.

Or perhaps you're someone who feels called to participate in the healing arts in some way on your own journey and you want to be part of a collective shared experience. Surely more of these opportunities will be presenting themselves as more people discover the potentiality of our current liminal spaces. If you put the intention out there, it will likely find you by synchronicity when you're receptive to the experience. Layer by layer, we work our way through to come out the other side.

CHAPTER 17

BUILDING RESILIENCE

Personal and Societal Regeneration

When we are stuck repeating old patterns in relationships and life, it's because the past is unresolved. It's like getting caught in a loop. This happens after painful life experiences that we couldn't digest and process in the moment.

We don't usually realize what we're carrying with us or how we're participating in it. We just see the repetition of the story that keeps replaying in different faces and places, causing more pain.

The unresolved past gets frozen in the body and subconscious until we can digest and process it. What has happened since 2020 is still frozen in all of us as individuals. It's also frozen in the collective consciousness. Now we are invited to thaw it out and discover the hidden gifts.

The land holds energy from what took place there, so naturally there are certain places on the planet where the COVID trauma grid is more intense based on the local history.

This might sound strange at first. So, think about a place where something scary or painful happened to you. Maybe you avoided it entirely, or for a while, so you could give yourself space to heal. If you went back again, maybe you could still feel it in the energy of the place.

It probably evoked visceral feelings about what happened there. Maybe you've also traveled to sites around the planet with an intense history and you sensed it, smelled it, or somehow felt it viscerally.

As we process and integrate our own past, the land clears as well because we've transmuted a pocket of energy in the local grid from suffering to resilience. Our personal integration process also has this healing effect on the collective consciousness. This is how the individual participates in healing society and our world. Likewise, our personal and ancestral unresolved past contributes to the collective burden. The issues we see in the world are the sum of our personal and generational baggage.

The ongoing existential crises unfolding in our world and in our personal lives are creating inner conflicts or dilemmas causing this stuff to surface and be felt. It has a unique flavor for each person based on our own unresolved past. Emotions and feelings come up that remind us of experiences from our history. This usually happens without our awareness, so naturally we react from our programming instead of making conscious choices.

When something shocking happens, that can spark new awareness and a sudden perspective shift. It can force us to see something we didn't notice or an option we hadn't considered before.

Many of us have been feeling called to a deeper questioning of life's meaning and purpose following the unexpected, shocking, and disorienting events of recent years. This is part of the gift. When we can recognize our limitations through the triggers of current experiences, we have the opportunity to liberate ourselves from captivity and to expand.

Similar to what happens to an abuse victim, the existentially shattering experiences in our world affect every aspect of human life: family, friends, intimate relationships, isolation and connection, work and career, finances, identity, values, beliefs, worldview, self-worth, meaning and purpose, freedom and responsibility, mental and physical health, spiritual awakening, life and death, connection with All That Is.

We've each been invited to focus more deeply on specific areas that affected us personally. Have you noticed particular patterns in your life?

When the past is unresolved, there's no real future. That is our biggest challenge. History repeats itself when everything is merely an unconscious repetition of the past trying to resolve itself, in escalating octaves until it gets our attention and we make new choices. Without awareness of our captivity in those patterns and the willingness to make new choices, it leads to more of the same.

The choice to emerge and evolve from the state of captivity is ours. As each of us does the inner work, we are also bringing peace to our ancestors and digesting parts of the collective trauma as well as clearing the Earth grids. This opens a path of light for humanity and future generations.

Emerging into resilience is our calling. This is an opportunity to awaken to who we really are, individually and as the human species. The more we resist this evolutionary process, the more we will suffer. We will be continually nudged to awaken and transform, personally and collectively, in increasingly more intense ways.

Developing resilience

Resilience is about adapting and bouncing back from tragedy, trauma, threats, significant stress, loss, and adversity. It means embodying greater wellbeing so we can share our gifts with the world. Resilience is one of the most important qualities and skills to master in the 2020s.

Resilience is a process, not a fixed state or destination. It's about *feeling the feels* while keeping going. Resilience does not come from avoidance, denial, or bypassing. It involves continually cultivating greater energy, presence, embodiment, and fluidity.

Resilience is not the same as surviving or simply enduring suffering. Surviving means you're alive but still *in it*—the frustration, scarcity, self-pity, dread, grief, anger, sadness, and other heavy emotions. In the suffering of mere survival, you don't see a way out, and it might even seem normal.

In the state of suffering, we often want to commiserate with others who are suffering. If you stay in it, you may survive it, but you'll pass that legacy to the next generation, which will have similar themes of struggle and suffering.

We inherited, from those who came before us, both the unresolved trauma as well as the resilience.

Resilience is about feeling, digesting, processing, and integrating the learning as wisdom and strength so that you can pass that gift on. As you do the inner work, you're making it easier for others to tune into your codes of resilience and feel inspired to transform their life.

The self-healing process is first about empowering yourself through self-honesty and a commitment to self-responsibility. Those are the pre-requisites for rebuilding self-worth, doing the inner work of growing up, and regenerating resilience. Then, layer by layer, you can *presence* and digest the unresolved emotional residue as well as continually updating your subconscious programming and identity.

The process becomes a gradual and increasing liberation of your soul, allowing you to discover your true self, expand into your higher potential, and live your unique divine purpose. Everyone and everything has a purpose.

The rest is just our programming, defense mechanisms, and automaton behavior. That's not the true self. But we identify with it because it's what we've known.

It's what's been done throughout human history because we didn't know any better. We are now living in times of new energies and expanded awareness, which means we can choose a different path than those who came before us.

Holistic resilience is key

The holistic dimension of resilience involves cultivating resilience on all levels of human life—physical, mental, emotional, financial, social, spiritual, and technological.

This is about creating a new dialogue among the past, present, and future. Instead of the past traumas determining who we are and who we can become, we can transform the past into a tool by transmuting it into resilience, which is a valuable resource for shaping the present and future.

Holistic resilience also involves exploring your ancestral resilience to connect with the innate strengths and wisdom that you inherited through your lineage so you can share your gifts and learning with others.

Your ancestors had difficult life experiences, too. Their unresolved trauma was passed on, and so was the resilience. For many of us, that legacy involves more trauma than resilience. We can change that now, as the generational curse-breakers, ending the old cycle and passing on a new legacy.

We can't bypass the healing by simply skipping ahead to the good parts or *just moving on*. Building resilience is a process, and it takes time, but it doesn't have to be as hard as you might think.

Early in the healing journey, we start setting new boundaries and saying no when something is not aligned with our values and goals. In fact, the first stages are mostly about what we are saying no to, internally and externally.

We start removing toxic people and habits of our own. We identify negative thought patterns and start talking to ourselves differently. We stop reacting to life in the same ways as before. We quit investing in what leads us away from the path of empowerment, healing, growth, liberation, and expansion.

Later in the healing journey, we start integrating much more of the good stuff. By then we are growing up enough to be able to hold the nuance instead of getting stuck in black-and-white thinking. We can recognize that we don't want to be like those who harmed us, and we no longer allow ourselves to participate in self-harm through toxic relationships and situations or self-sabotage behaviors—*and* we can recognize the gems of wisdom and gifts of virtues that we can extract from the rubble.

You're not the same person you were in 2020. Likewise, you're not the same person you were before an abusive relationship or situation. You're not the same person you were last year.

As transformational leadership psychologist Dr. Benjamin Hardy says in his rapid transformation trainings: "You're not even the same person you were at breakfast this morning."

Have you noticed what's different about who you are today compared to five years ago? Ten years ago? Pause and reflect on that a bit.

Hardy often refers to "psychological flexibility" as our ability to re-frame our past and our identity as we continually grow and change. He says this is key for personal development and rapid transformation. Hardy also encourages us to check in with ourselves frequently: "Who are you being accountable to right now—your past self or your future self?"

We can add more dimensions to this same concept by shifting it into the realm of *holistic flexibility*. This is what is needed to build holistic resilience.

Essentially, holistic resilience is about strengthening the human spirit and bringing that into every aspect of our lives during challenging times on planet Earth.

Embodiment starts the process

After trauma it's common to dissociate, zone out, or check out of the body. Over time, this becomes a mind–body split, an inner separation. Typically, the body will get most neglected because it's easier to escape pain through the mind. It's helpful to practice embodiment to reconnect with your whole self.

Embodiment is the practice where healing becomes lived. Trauma fragments our sense of self, safety, and belonging. Integration begins not just by understanding what happened and talking about it, but by returning to the body as the place where presence can be restored.

Embodiment invites us to feel again, safely and gradually in order to process our feelings, so we can metabolize what was once frozen and exiled. It's a process of befriending the body instead of running away from it or trying to control it. Through embodiment, the body becomes a vehicle of truth, not just survival. In this space, we begin to create the roots for our healing, not just as an idea but as a lived, visceral reality.

It might not have felt safe to be in your body during traumatic events. So, retraining yourself to return to center could be challenging because your subconscious and nervous system may sense danger. This is usually based on a memory that feels like it's happening now because we are vividly remembering it.

The easiest way to reconnect with your body is through your breath and *presencing*. This focused awareness practice will allow you to observe what's emerging from your body without trying to fix anything. Embodiment helps you to give yourself permission to be fully present with what wants to emerge into awareness. It sounds so simple, yet committing to this daily practice will start to transform your life in *big* ways!

I would suggest you find a comfortable, safe spot where you can do this practice intentionally. In nature it's amazing, especially when you're barefoot or sitting on the earth. But that might not be possible, or feel safe, for everyone. So maybe for you it's a patio chair or meditation cushion inside your home.

Close your eyes and focus your awareness on your breath as you inhale through the nose and exhale through the mouth. As you continue inhaling through the nose and exhaling through the mouth, with each breath, allow your awareness to settle down into your body as your body settles down into the chair.

Continue breathing naturally and becoming more present with yourself. Notice what's showing up for you in the moment. Maybe certain sensations, feelings, or parts of your body. Allow yourself to notice without trying to fix it, change it, judge it, reject it, or analyze it. Just allow it to emerge and be seen, heard, felt, and held with compassion and the light of your awareness. You might want to journal about your insights after your experience.

When you sign up for my newsletter on my homepage, www.innerintegration.com you get access to my free guided meditation to walk you through this process called the Daily Embodiment Practice.

Resolving the past to create a new future

Resolved means we can feel it, digest it, process it, and integrate the learning.

First, it's essential to feel it—thawing out layer by layer, the ugly and uncomfortable feelings that were frozen in the nervous system and buried in the subconscious so we could keep surviving and doing life. This is where your embodiment practice comes in.

It might sound scary to feel this stuff because you might be afraid to get stuck in the feelings. But it's possible to feel it without getting stuck in it.

Next, we digest it.

During digestion, the mouth and stomach break things down into bite-sized pieces. This is when we communicate, journal, and analyze what happened.

We'll often ruminate during this part of the process, but we don't want to get stuck where worries and food stagnation in the stomach start to cause digestive issues. When things stagnate in rumination, it's usually because we are stuck in a victim story trying to figure out what happened. Listen to the way you're framing the story in your inner dialogue and notice where you can empower yourself through self-responsibility.

Next, the small intestine separates the nutrients from the waste. We don't want to discard everything from the food of our experiences. Nutrients are important and will be used to form new life, becoming cells, blood, organs, and all the systems of the body. Likewise, we can filter out the important nutrients from our painful experiences, extracting the gifts of wisdom, strength, learning, and resilience among other virtues.

The body gets rid of the waste; likewise, we don't have to hold on to all the stuff that no longer serves us from the painful experiences of our past. And so, we continue processing.

The large intestine will gather any remaining nutrients as the waste continues to get removed. Some of it is easier to release. Sometimes some of the grief becomes constipated and takes longer to work its way out because we are holding on. Some things are more challenging to let go of.

Digestion allows us to process and integrate the learning of our experiences, layer by layer. This is how we alchemize the past into gold. Then it becomes the resilience we pass on to the next generation.

When the past is resolved, there's space for a new consciousness to enter. Clearing the emotional residue creates space for the new—new ideas, insights, responses, solutions, perspectives, possibilities, relationships, and experiences. We don't have to know all the answers and solutions. First, we create the space for the new to emerge.

Legacy repurposing

Our ancestors lived through many traumas. Because they survived, we are here now. Yet much of their trauma was not resolved and became the burden passed on to us. We also inherited the resilience of our ancestors—the gifts of their strength and wisdom that they transmuted from their own challenges.

Likewise, we will either pass on the legacy of the unresolved, undigested trauma or we will pass on a legacy of resilience. Truth be told, it will be a mix of both, but it can either be trauma-heavy or resilience-light. This is our choice as individuals and our individual choices become the collective human path.

If we do not step up for ourselves in big ways now during these pivotal times in human history, the future of humanity will not be bright.

While many of us are already aware of some of the harm caused to the youngest generations during the COVID measures, such as reduced IQ and increased mental illness, we have no idea of the long-term repercussions of that never-done-before social experiment when their key developmental years were interrupted and stunted.

While it may sound logical to focus on healing the kids, I would suggest first, *parent, heal thyself.*

In working with clients, I've observed how adults transmute something from the darkness into light, and that change is instantly mirrored in their kids who are under seven or eight years old. The parents are usually surprised they didn't even have to explain anything to their kids. *It just happened.*

That's because the kids were tuned into one frequency through the parent, then they automatically shifted into a new frequency when the parent shifted. It's like changing the TV channel from the old legacy of trauma to the new legacy of light.

This process usually takes longer with older kids because they have more layers of trauma and defense mechanisms, but it's still wild to see the subtle shifts occurring in adult kids as the parents make their own inner shifts.

Maybe you're thinking, that's great, but I don't have kids so what's the point? Each of us affects the world around us, whether we have kids or not. Every day we interact with others and transfer darkness by reacting to each other's trauma, or we share light codes.

As you heal yourself, you're also bringing peace to your ancestors. We can offer healing to our ancestors when we transmute layers of the darkness into light. That clearing sends ripple effects through the morphogenic field of the DNA to all our ancestors who want to tune into the new light codes. Even if you don't have kids, you have cousins in the human race that you've never even met because the further back we go, the closer we all are.

Most of the clients I've worked with are the adult kids taking on this massive responsibility to clear their lineage after generations of abuse and neglect. Sometimes I get to work with the parents and grandparents who realize they passed on the legacy of trauma unintentionally. It's much easier for the kids when the parent heals first. Blessed are the kids whose parents are taking on the responsibility of doing their inner healing work, and brighter is their future because of it.

So here we are at this pivotal opportunity in human history to hear the calling and step up as individuals, whether we have kids or not, to contribute to a better world for future generations as well as bringing peace to ourselves and our ancestors. Our actions are changing our relationship with the past, present, and future.

The answer to fixing the world is not outside ourselves—it is within. When we are focused externally, we are avoiding our inner work.

So, if we want to see a healing world, first we create the space for the new to emerge by resolving the past and integrating the trauma within ourselves. Have faith in the ripple effect. Your contribution matters. *You* matter.

Self-healing contributes to collective healing. Each of us affects the whole of humanity. The more of us who are doing this inner work, the faster and easier others can heal because they'll have access to our light codes.

This is how we build resilience and open a path of light for humanity and future generations. It's the process of repurposing our legacy and passing on the resilience, backward and forward in time.

In my Legacy Repurposing group coaching program, I help people to transform their wounds into a legacy of light, as an artist uses unwanted or discarded materials to create something new and meaningful.

In art, repurposing involves infusing new narratives and perspectives into materials that have lost their original purpose or value. It's a way of creating new communication among the past, present, and future.

This holistic transformational process is similar. *You are the artist of your life*. Your deepest wounds can become your greatest gifts when you repurpose the internal materials (emotions, feelings, ideas, beliefs, identities, and memories of past experiences, as well as those you inherited through your genetic lineage) by giving them new function and meaning. This allows you to emerge renewed, with a deeper and evolving understanding of who you are and what your divine purpose is in the world.

Each of us has a unique purpose and higher potential waiting to be discovered and actualized. We can use creativity and art as powerful transformative tools for trauma healing and personal evolution.

As we unearth the roots of our personal and ancestral history, these can be planted in new, amended soil where they'll be nourished to create something beautiful, purposeful, joyful, and abundant. This is the process of regenerating resilience.

CHAPTER 18

ACTIVE IMAGINATION

Your Greatest Power

As we navigate the raw possibilities inherent in liminality, we are faced with the potential to create the life we really want to live. Our future as individuals and society depends on what we do with the extraordinary evolutionary opportunity we are being presented with during the 2020s.

Your active imagination is your greatest tool for transforming your life. It is your God-given birthright to use the power of your imagination to create the life you want to live. Yet this power ought to be wielded responsibly and in alignment with divine will.

The *beings without conscience inhabited by evil entities acting good* know all about this secret—in fact, they're using it against us.

In a state of captivity and the defense mechanisms caused by trauma—fight, flight, fear, freeze, collapse, denial, defense, or dissociation—your active imagination is not accessible. Instead, you're on automaton mode, defaulting to your programming, which is like a passive form of imagination that's creating all the things you don't want.

Have you ever noticed how your mind can automatically imagine the worst-case scenarios when you're in a state of fear? Or how you might read some awful news, then start imagining what it would be like if that were happening to you? None of that is what you want, but when we are passively imagining the worst, we are giving power to it unintentionally.

Intention is the key to active imagination.

They need us to participate in "re-imagining global society," a concept that was introduced during COVID. There are organizations now dedicated to this campaign, of course, using lots of euphemisms that make it sound good.

When we are passively imagining, we are unknowingly misusing our power to create the world of global governance that *they* want. *They* cannot do it without us. The same is true in any abusive relationship or smaller social system.

We can choose to unsubscribe as much as possible from all the noxious influences that aim to keep us infantilized, sick, defensive, disconnected, dysfunctional, overwhelmed, and disempowered. To do so, we will need to consciously tap into our imagination and use it wisely.

Most of us have never been taught to train ourselves to use our active imagination to create the life we want to live. Children are often tapped into the creative power of imagination. However, many of us were told by teachers or parents, "It's just your imagination."

The interesting thing is that our consciousness is more powerful than all the social-engineering and trauma-based mind control. We've been tricked into giving our power away to that stuff, which makes us feel victimized, powerless, helpless, and apathetic because it feels like there's no escape. We've been taught lies that keep us playing small, dimming our light, settling for less than we are worth, and living in a state of captivity.

It's wild how fast things can change when we shift state and tap into this inner power. If more of us could do this, we would be living in a *very* different world. That would not take nearly as long as you might think.

Your state of consciousness matters

When you're in a low-frequency state, such as guilt, shame, fear, grief, despair, or anger, you're a prime target for parasites and predators in the physical and spiritual world. This is how trauma often begets more trauma. In these states, you don't have access to your higher human consciousness faculties.

When you're in a higher state of consciousness, you have access to courage, discernment, love, creativity, imagination, insight, and intuition. These are necessary for thriving as human beings.

Thriving is the later stage of healing, expanding into self-actualization. Unfortunately, we can't just skip to this stage. When we attempt to do so, we will continually get triggered back into states of victimhood to review and process the unresolved trauma.

Lower and higher states of consciousness are not about blame or judgment. They are a measure of frequency. You can look up images of the scale of human consciousness and the book *Power vs. Force* by David Hawkins.

Of course *they* want us in an immobilized, collapsed, powerless, and wounded inner child state characterized by fawning and compliance, dissociation, feeling hopeless, overwhelmed, in despair, lost, alone, insecure, and dependent, or in a destructive self-sabotaging adolescent state where we use adaptations, such as defensiveness, destruction and self-destruction, aggression, self-righteousness, avoidance, suppression, and addictions. In those triggered states we give away our power and are easy to control by outside forces.

When we don't have access to our healthy, responsible adult state or higher self, everything else falls apart from there—relationships, families, communities, communication, physical and mental health, work performance, wealth and abundance, growth, healing, focus, self-worth, self-esteem, self-care, self-trust, self-love, critical thinking, intuition, insight, imagination, creativity, authenticity, and purpose.

It's the same in abusive relationships. Abusers take down every pillar of a target's life by keeping the target in a low state of consciousness. The overt ones do it directly. The covert ones do it insidiously and meticulously, even getting you to do it to yourself.

They don't have to destroy our lives. *They* can get us to destroy ourselves, which makes their work a lot easier. Keeping us in a low state of consciousness is how the few control the many. As we do the inner work, we gain new access to higher states of consciousness, including the power of our imagination to create the world we actually want to live in.

There's a scene from the movie *The NeverEnding Story*, when Atreyu confronts G'mork. The dialog reveals *exactly* what's happening in a society in which people have collapsed into despair and emptiness:

> G'mork: People have begun to lose their hopes and forget their dreams. So the Nothing grows stronger.
>
> Atreyu: What is the Nothing?
>
> G'mork: It's the emptiness that's left. It's like a despair destroying this world. And I have been trying to help it.
>
> Atreyu: But why?
>
> G'mork: Because people who have no hopes are easy to control; and whoever has the control...has the power![82]

Something like *the Nothing* is also taking over our world. But all is not lost.

In the movie, it's the power of dreams, creativity, and imagination that manifests a beautiful world again, bringing new light and life to what was dark, destroyed, and disappearing.

However, we can't access the state of positive imagination and creativity when we are triggered into states of the wounded and self-destructive inner child.

When the defense system is activated, the safe and social system is offline, and so is the rest and digest function. The nervous system is binary. That means the activation of the defense system locks us out of our ability to connect and co-regulate with others, to return to homeostasis for optimal health, as well as our ability to access higher states of consciousness. That's why it's so important to do the inner work of transmuting the darkness into light.

Creativity is the antidote to destruction.

The two balancing forces in our universe are creativity and destruction, and we are undoubtedly living in times of the collapse and destruction of old systems. Those structures and systems aren't working anymore because the energy is shifting and more of us are awakening.

Our consciousness can no longer maintain the old corrupt system, so it is imploding. A new world is certainly emerging this decade, but what kind of world depends on how we respond to these challenges, and whether we take our power back and liberate ourselves.

What happened in the past, and what's happening right now, as evil is running rampant in our world, doesn't have to be the future that we create. We can rise to the calling and step up in bigger ways for ourselves, our families, communities, and the future of humanity.

You have a higher potential waiting to be discovered and actualized as you clear away the residue from the past, restore wholeness to your soul, and integrate the resilience such as the wisdom and strength. You can use the power of creativity and art as transformative tools for personal and ancestral trauma healing and evolution. Together we can imagine and create a much more harmonious world in which humans, this planet, and all species we cohabitate with can thrive.

The power of imagination

I invite you to explore a new creative ritual for bedtime. This is what Neville Goddard referred to as the "imaginal state," which was the core of his work with manifestation.

Goddard learned from his guide and then taught others about the power of imagination to transform lives. He taught that the most powerful time to tap into this inner resource is right before falling asleep.

What you're thinking about and feeling in the moments before falling asleep is carried into your subconscious while you sleep. The next day, and the following days and weeks, you see those themes in your life. Most of us aren't paying attention to this. We are often watching the news, movies, scrolling online, or thinking about our problems and everything we have to do until we doze off, allowing those influences to program our subconscious. This is passive imagination.

If you interrupt the process of passive imagination and do the imaginal state practice intentionally, you will start to notice how uncanny it is, which will help you to recognize the power that you have to transform your life.

Of course, I want to reiterate the importance of aligning your will with divine will. God will sometimes let you manifest things you're not ready for or that aren't good for you so that you can explore those desires and learn. Ultimately everything will crash and collapse unless you realize where it's heading and humble yourself first. That's why you'll hear stories of people who manifested massive things and then lost it all.

So, when you're practicing active imagination and using the power of the imaginal state to manifest the life you want to live, be sure to ask yourself what your intention is for that manifestation, as well as asking your higher power if that's the most aligned path for you. I also want to reiterate the importance of doing the inner work and not bypassing your unresolved trauma by jumping straight to manifestation. There's a reason this is the *last* chapter of the book.

Have you ever noticed how the darkness tries to creep into your thoughts and feeling state as you're falling asleep or how it sometimes wakes you up in the middle of the night with anxiety or night terrors? In those moments, it's the most challenging to remember your power and re-direct your mind to imagine what you want in your life.

Remind yourself when you lay down at night to consciously start choosing your thoughts, your state, and what you're allowing into your awareness. Negative thoughts will elicit heavy emotions and feelings. Positive thoughts will make you feel good and optimistic.

Carefully consider what you're exposing yourself to, both internally and externally, as you're falling asleep. It's not the best time to read or watch the news and other toxic influences in videos, movies, or series. Don't fall asleep listening to something like that because the subliminal messages are going directly into your subconscious while you're sleeping.

When you first start this new practice, right away you'll probably notice how many negative thoughts based on worry, anxiety, doubt, and fear come up as you're trying to imagine what you want to create. That's normal, so don't beat yourself up about it. If you hear those thoughts, cancel or delete them immediately. Then redirect yourself to what you want to create in your life. Remember, the more of your unresolved trauma that you process and integrate, the easier it will be for you to stay in an empowered state and manifest what is aligned with your divine mission and highest timeline.

If you're being interrupted by thoughts about tasks you need to do during waking hours, write those down so you don't have to keep wasting your energy trying to remember them all.

If you're interrupted by invasive thoughts of distorted desires, you can declare new decisions, such as, "I repent for harboring wrath toward people who hurt me," or "I repent for allowing myself to get swept away into lust." You can also declare things like, "I release myself from the obligation of internalizing my family's feelings," or "I release myself from the obligation of carrying my abuser's shame."

If fear is overpowering you, you can declare something like, "I rebuke the spirit of fear. I repent for believing that I have to do it all on my own. I am opening my heart to the Creator and remembering that I'm not alone in this world because the Creator has my back."

Allow yourself to imagine what you're creating with all your senses, as if it's already happened. Imagine that what you really want has already become your new normal. Notice how the little and big things start aligning in your life with your creative imagination visualizations. Amazing things are happening for you!

This is a practice you can do all day long. It's the most powerful right before you fall asleep because your brain is already entering into alpha and theta brainwave states, giving you access to the subconscious.

Your subconscious can't tell the difference between what you're vividly imagining and what's actually happening. That can work against us when we are in a low state of consciousness, such as the state of captivity. Or we can use this power in a higher state of consciousness to create our dreams.

Imagination is your most powerful tool to transform your reality, though it can work positively or negatively for you depending on your intention and awareness as well as where you are in your healing journey.

Keep canceling the negative, fear-based thoughts and redirect them to the positive. If you're talking poorly about yourself, unsubscribe from those lies and remind yourself how worthy and capable you are.

Before doing imagination practices, shift into a state of gratitude and faith that amazing things are happening for you. This is easier said than done. When you're in the middle of fear oppression, it's challenging to remember that you have the power to shift your state. There are some helpful videos on YouTube from various creators if you search for "amazing things are happening to me."

Fear is evil's greatest weapon against humanity and that's why fear is the currency of control in abusive relationships, families, workplaces, communities, and society. Remember, this is all emotional manipulation and spiritual oppression. *They* are trying to trick us into consenting to being used as energy sources to create that fear-based world because it feeds them and makes them feel powerful. But *they* can't create it without us. *They* are aware of our power, and *they* desperately don't want us to discover it.

Worrying is the dark art of using the imagination to create something you don't want. We've all been there, on default mode, because that is our ancestral programming.

When we consciously create through active imagination, we can stop participating in the world *they* want by investing our power and resources in a different direction. Imagine the world that *you* want to live in and pass on to future generations.

It doesn't mean ignoring reality. If we ignore what's happening in our world and personal lives, if we ignore our unresolved trauma, we will end up denying, bypassing, and avoiding the issues, which leads to further trauma, victimization, and harm.

It's not black and white—it's nuanced. Can you pay attention to what's happening around and within you without giving your power away to it *and* imagine the life you want to live?

When you're planting seeds in the garden, you don't dig them up to check on them. You nurture the soil and let nature do its thing. Likewise, *how* your dreams manifest isn't your concern. The universe will rearrange itself to match your assumptions. Your job is to actively imagine and hold the state of faith that it's inevitable because worthiness and creativity is your divine birthright.

Discovering the power of our imagination means we can step into a more authentic version of who we really are. From this state, we can create the greatest benefit for ourselves and the future of humanity.

CONCLUSION

WHY IT MATTERS

The state of captivity is the predicament of our time. Perhaps it always has been, in one way or another, during the course of human history. However, this is not our true nature. As more people are waking up, empowering and liberating ourselves, we are shifting the trajectory of ourselves and our species.

In some ways, we have come a long way. More people are becoming aware of the existence of evil and the prevalence of abuse in their personal lives and in society. Yet most of humanity is still disempowered and in a state of victimhood.

Right now, we are being ushered faster than we realize into a whole other level of captivity. Our unresolved past is being uploaded to technology and AI, which is going to mirror and magnify it in unimaginable ways.

In the very near future, our world will become unrecognizable. Along the way, we will be presented with invitations to give up more of our autonomy, sovereignty, and freedom. If we learn from the past, we can expect that these invitations will involve promises *for our own good* and *for the greater good.*

Fear bombardment campaigns will be dosed with acts of perceived kindness. There will be attempts to further isolate us, physically and psychologically. And there will be a perceived inability to escape the pull into it all. Technology will be presented as a savior from the chaos and collapse of our current global, local, and personal problems.

Of course, technology and AI offer some amazing benefits to make human life easier and better. Yet what matters is how we use it. If we want to move forward in a positive direction, it's vital that we learn from our mistakes and recognize this calling to heal our personal and ancestral traumas, lest we drift into the next frontier of captivity as we did during the COVID campaign.

During the COVID years, we witnessed the potent combination of fear appeals with messages of hope, leading to about 80 percent of the world complying with the measures. Without a public conversation about what happened and how we participated, without publicly acknowledging the crimes against humanity that took place, without some kind of reckoning about the unresolved past, we will likely repeat it because we haven't learned from it.

I hope this book has inspired you to gain new insights into your personal experiences and what you witnessed on the collective level. Perhaps you also feel motivated to empower yourself, to do the inner work and regenerate resilience, so that you can thrive, no matter the chaos happening out there as we navigate these liminal spaces between worlds.

When you feel stuck and don't know what to do, ask yourself how it's serving you. Keep coming back to this question when you hear your mind wanting to go into the victim consciousness of powerlessness, helplessness, and apathy. As you digest the past, integrate yourself from a state of fragmentation into a state of wholeness and reprogram your subconscious to focus on creating positive solutions, it will stop trying to fix your life through self-sabotage.

I believe the ongoing existential pressure is a transformational calling to those who are here to envision and build a new world, transmuting the darkness into light and leading the way for humanity as we emerge from the liminal spaces following the global crises of the 2020s.

The overall theme of the coming years is *the unexpected*. Many people are sensing the discomfort of the unknown on the horizon. We used to talk about our five-year plans, our ten-year plans, and what we plan to do in retirement. This is more challenging now as none of us has any idea what our world will look like in just a few years.

We will be pushed to re-think our collective systems and the way individuals exist within the collective. It's no longer about the old ways of losing one's self through unity or conformity with society. It's also no longer about the selfish, self-centered individual who doesn't care about the rest. At this stage of human evolution, it's now becoming the era of the authentic, sovereign, empowered, liberated individual within the collective who voluntarily contributes to the collective.

Big and relevant questions are surfacing about how humans and AI will co-exist and what that means for us all.

We will likely see technological advancements that will either serve individuals and humanity or aim to imprison us in captivity—and probably a bit of both.

We will either see the emergence of more humanitarian systems that make life easier for us as individuals and a society, or next-level abusive systems disguised as *for the collective good*—and probably a bit of both.

The more technology advances, what's real becomes ever more confusing, especially online. Energetic discernment will be one of the most important life skills for these times. The shifts in our world require us to be able to sense frequency and recognize its nature vibrationally.

For the past several hundred years, humans have been most reliant on logic, mental processing, reason, and external validation. Certainly, the mind is a fantastic human trait that animals don't have access to. Yet our true power does not come from the mind. Perhaps it is simply impeccable divine timing that our sense of mental certainty is being stripped away by the unprecedented changes in our world.

The mind is not our best tool for discernment. Many things are disguised, appearing as one thing, but are actually something else. The mind sometimes can't tell the difference, especially when it gets caught up in distractions, expectations, rationalizations, distorted desires, fantasies, and other forms of mental masturbation.

Those who are mind-centered will struggle through these shifts. The more we grasp onto rigid rules and obsolete perceptions of certainty, the more we will struggle. The more confused we are about what's real, the more susceptible we are to deception. The more we hold on to victim consciousness, the more we will suffer in powerlessness and poverty of the soul.

Human Design is a fascinating system that weaves together modern science, such as quantum physics and genetics with ancient wisdom, such as astrology, the I Ching and the chakra system. It's like a cosmic blueprint that reveals how we are wired to make decisions, interact with the world, and express our life purpose. This self-knowledge can be helpful for understanding our strengths and challenges so we can live in more effortless alignment with our true selves. There are personal and collective applications. According to Human Design, as we start moving into the next evolution of human consciousness in 2027, our primary awareness center and seat of decision-making is going to be the solar plexus, which governs intuition, emotional clarity, true self, and spiritual discernment. We will find our power in the choices we make from these aspects, not from the logical mind.

This is precisely why the dark forces of our world, from the micro level to the macro level, are trying to confuse us, put us in a brain fog, make us more defensive and dysfunctional, disconnected from each other as well as severed from our connection with All That Is. These circumstances condition us into a state of learned helplessness where we outsource our power and perception of reality. Yet they are also pushing us to evolve.

We can already see the new awareness shifting in humanity.

Those who were guided solely by mental constructs, looking for external validation, basing the perception of reality and decision-making on logic, rules, societal expectations, *expertology*, and "peer-reviewed studies" during the mass deception of the COVID campaign were led astray into a false perception of reality, which they were coerced into believing was so certain and real. They were driven by fear, self-preservation, and societal pressure to gain the false security of external validation.

Those who were able to tap into the solar plexus awareness could feel that something was off. We used our emotional clarity, intuition, and spiritual discernment to decipher what was real and what wasn't, to make choices that support our health, sanity, and wellbeing, even when we didn't necessarily have the rational facts to back it up. It doesn't mean we didn't have any fear, but when we did, we stood by our principles, even when the peer pressure was overwhelming. We just *sensed* what we needed to do.

We can't be lied to and deceived as easily when we have the emotional clarity and discernment of solar plexus awareness. However, this clarity depends on how clear the solar plexus is.

Try as the manipulators might to censor the truth and spread confusing propaganda from all angles, when we have clear solar plexus awareness, we can sense the vibration of lies and feel the truth in our body, even when we don't have external proof yet.

The movie *The Matrix* depicted how humans were being used as energy sources and organic batteries for the inorganic machine-like rulers of our world, which is a fantastic metaphor for the *beings without conscience inhabited by evil entities playing good* a.k.a. psychopaths—a mental construct term which doesn't fully explain their nature or what they do in this world.

The matrix is a construct of the mind, like a giant holographic spider web entangling and influencing the psyche of humans, even from far ends of the construct.

When we own the clarity and power of our solar plexus emotional awareness, we are no longer offering our emotions to be harvested for feeding the distorted power structures of this world, which use it all against us.

That doesn't mean we don't have blinds pots. Our blind spots are any areas of unresolved trauma and emotional residue distorting our perception of reality, of self as well as our desires.

The global mafia are rushing to push through their Grand Finale of a power grab during this decade. They know that their reign of centuries of mind control over humanity is ending unless they find a way to hack our bodies with technology to override our innate divine wisdom.

They will make plenty of mistakes by way of hubris. Likewise, we can fall into a similar trap because pride is just a distorted desire coming from an ego-based inferiority/superiority stance.

Resolving trauma is essential for having a clear channel of solar plexus awareness. Emotional processing is the key to making this quantum leap in human evolution without having to struggle so much. When we are overloaded with mental distortions and emotional residue from past traumas, we don't have clear access to intuition and solar plexus emotional discernment.

What I'm seeing on the macro level, I also see with my work in trauma integration. Every time I guide clients into their body to track the imprint of their core wound, they almost always find it in their "stomach," which is the solar plexus area. The sensations of the wound tend to radiate outward to other areas, which are often more noticeable first, but the epicenter of the unresolved trauma is usually in the solar plexus.

It's no coincidence that we are living in times of increasing trauma.

On the one hand, this is overwhelming. On the other hand, it's triggering our unresolved trauma—including the ancestral trauma we inherited—so that these can enter our awareness, then be processed and integrated so we can evolve as individuals and humanity.

It's also no coincidence that we have been conditioned to be ever more reliant on external validation and mental constructs of reality that are coming from the media, social media, and other virtual spaces.

It's becoming more challenging to distinguish truth from illusion. That stress is causing people to outsource their perception of reality in exchange for a sense of relief. It's also causing people to become more dependent on external validation for a sense of security.

With so many emotionally charged narratives being spun from every direction, we are being desensitized, or hyper-sensitized, both of which distort our pure energetic sensitivity that allows us to be attuned to the subtle energies within ourselves and in the world around us.

The old collective systems that humans built from mental constructs are going to continue breaking down so we can create and adapt to new ways of living. The challenge is that we will be susceptible to rescue fantasies and promises of convenience or security if we allow ourselves to outsource our inner authority.

On the interpersonal and the societal level, it's not about the individual vs. the collective. It's about the authenticity, empowerment, and liberation of individuals *within* the collective, which benefits and brings harmony to both. It's important to remember this as things escalate in the coming years.

The shifts in our world are bringing changes to our intimate relationships as well—the smallest unit of the human collective.

We are shifting out of the era of codependent and role-based relationships into higher vibrational partnerships based on mutual self-awareness, responsibility, sovereignty, co-creation, and a shared divine mission while both partners are living from a sense of inner purpose and personal fulfillment, which leads to shared healing, growth, liberation, and evolution.

It's not a coincidence that the biggest challenge for relationships nowadays is the emotional realm. When two people meet, it's often more like trauma meets trauma, which leads to more trauma, defensiveness, dysfunction, and disconnection.

This is why so many relationships fail and people are seeking new ways of "connecting," most of which is unfortunately defensiveness coming from a place of unresolved trauma and leading to more trauma instead of true connection.

Many people are trying to connect through externally imposed mental constructs instead of from what's real, because that's what we are conditioned to chase and be. When the facade breaks down, the emotional residue from unresolved trauma is quickly triggered. Then the mind makes up a (likely delusional) story about it instead of recognizing that there's an opportunity for learning, healing, and integration.

Integration is a sacred healing process. It's the return of what was once fragmented into coherent wholeness. It's not just psychological—it's also energetic, somatic and spiritual. Integration means letting the body release what it was holding in order to survive. It means allowing frozen emotions to thaw into presence. It's about welcoming back the parts of ourselves that had to go into hiding. Integration is about living from essence instead of defensive adaptation. It isn't about "getting over it" or "moving on." It's about *becoming whole.*

The more emotional residue that builds up from traumatic experiences, the more we tend to avoid or suppress it instead of processing and integrating, which then leads to more distortion, dysfunction, and disconnection.

Our ability to connect with others depends on our inner healing, the clearing of past emotional residue and conditioning, so that we can be more present, more empowered, and more able to process with greater ease in the moment. Then we can connect from a deeper place of authenticity, transparency, awareness, responsibility, freedom, and truth.

Healing our emotional trauma is the only way to access emotional clarity. Our awareness is being shifted into the solar plexus so we can access our power there. Yet it's hidden and distorted under the layers of unresolved trauma and emotional residue.

This is why there are so many symptoms of uncontrolled trauma in our world, and that trend will continue until we face it because this is our evolutionary calling during this time in human history.

As we navigate the transition between the old and new paradigms, we are in the liminal space of uncertainty, which is scary, yet it's also the opening to infinite possibility.

In this transitional state, there's a loosening of the grip of the old rigid systems and rules that are no longer working with the new energies. Resisting these changes and trying to hold onto the old ways will only lead to more struggle. Bringing in new technological systems that create the same old state of captivity will also lead to more suffering.

Emotional mastery is the key to accessing solar plexus discernment and ride the waves of emotion without making reactive, misled decisions. Clarity arises as the peaks and lows of emotional turbulence settle and we can make calm decisions from an inner place of peace.

Trauma integration is essential for releasing the social conditioning, subconscious programming, and emotional residue from the past. This includes processing the ongoing disruptions and sense of loss as the old systems collapse.

Creating new forms of inner safety and sovereignty will be essential for releasing our attachments and addictions to the outdated systems so we don't choose more of the same when it is offered to us via a rescue fantasy. With inner safety, we can let go of the false security blankets we used to rely on, which are now so worn and torn that they're falling apart at the seams.

Updating our frame of identity on an ongoing basis is the key to being able to release the limiting past narratives and paradigms about who we are so that we can step into higher potential and higher timelines. These timeline shifts are now starting to happen very suddenly. Much can change *on a quantum dime* in the new cosmic energies.

Discernment is essential to recognizing what feels authentic and aligned so that we can identify shared values and resonance in order to be guided toward the people, resources, and situations where we will be able to create and thrive during these times of big changes.

When everything is collapsing like a scene from the movie *Inception*, there's a temptation to drift into nihilism and depersonalization. If nothing feels real anymore, that's either a launching point toward transformation and growth, or insanity and apathy. Discernment will lead us through the heavy fog and the smoke and mirrors.

Embodiment is key to returning our locus of discernment and decision-making inward to strengthen our presence, awareness, and sovereignty from a grounded place instead of seeking false refuge in the constructs of the mind, or worse yet, dissociating entirely.

Holistic resilience is key to being able to continue navigating the chaos, extracting the gifts and adapting to the changes in our world so we can survive and thrive during these times.

Spiritual awakening and integration are essential for continually evolving as individuals and humanity so we can navigate technological development in responsible and beneficial ways. We will also need to fully integrate our spirituality with our humanity instead of avoiding or shunning the flesh and the totality of who we are. It's not about escaping our humanity via spiritual bypassing or ignoring the spiritual dimension entirely. It's about integrating the two.

Creative expression through artistic form is key to exploring beyond the rational mind, imagining and creating the world we want to live in and the life we want to manifest in the new world.

To sum up the transitions we are moving through on a personal and collective level during these times: We are navigating the liminal space between trauma and purpose.

We are being called to trust the evolutionary process and step bravely into the unknown as co-creators. The ongoing crises and the shift in human consciousness are inviting us to trust intuition, to explore with curiosity and an open mind the unfolding revelation of life.

For sure we will face more existential debates about the nature of humanity, our relationship with self and with each other, as well as with technology, including our place in this universe.

This is the start of the new world now. There's a powerful catalysis happening in aligned connections where we each shift in positive ways by sharing light codes with one another.

Yet this is only happening in connections where people are empowered—in a state of full self-responsibility. It's not happening when we are in victimhood. Those interactions are becoming more draining. In a state of victim consciousness, we aren't receptive to the light codes.

It's incredibly powerful when we transmute our darkness into light, not just in terms of how that transforms our own lives, but also how much more amplified this effect is when we share these codes together. This is happening through the solar plexus emotional awareness.

In a group setting of people who are sharing light codes, that effect is incredibly powerful!

This is why abusers use the divide-and-conquer tactic to keep us apart physically, ideologically, and through triggering one another's defense mechanisms due to unresolved trauma.

When we are in victimhood, we are blocked from sharing light codes. Even when one person is in a state of victim consciousness, there's a distortion in the quantum field that prevents the sharing and activation from happening. When we are in an internal state of empowerment, we are able to share light codes and activate one another.

We also need to be in a state of empowerment and responsibility to connect with others without triggering each other's defense mechanisms at a neurological level.

The perpetrators in our world know how powerful we are when we can truly connect and activate each other through frequency exposure. They're also very aware about the energetic shifts happening during this time. That's why they are vying so hard for total control of humanity in the 2020s.

They know that this will be their last stand because the shifting frequencies on our planet are boosting a critical mass to finally be able to break through the captivity. As we heal and integrate, we can share light codes and activate one another, amplifying our power through connection, creating a new world based on what's real and what matters instead of the old construct they created for us where we are easily entrapped.

The more of us who heal and activate and share our light codes, the easier it will be for others to shift out of the victim consciousness. Though not everyone will make that free will choice.

I know that many people are struggling now. The weight of the past several years of stress is piling up on top of the unresolved traumas everyone is carrying from long before.

I want to invite you to see that we are entering a new world now.

The quality of the energy is different and it's much easier to make quantum shifts out of old patterns and predicaments. What is vibrationally aligned for your future self is becoming much more of a "Heaven, yes!" or a "Hell, no!" Can you feel it?

You don't have to keep struggling. Life doesn't have to be so hard anymore. You can empower and liberate yourself from your past, as well as the ancestral trauma you inherited that was never really yours to begin with. If that's what you want.

The more you invest in your inner work, the easier you will flow with the evolutionary energies of these times.

I'm sensing that much more craziness will happen in the world, and you might be, too. Yet that will continue to wake more people up, much like in abusive relationships. We can create our own little frequency bubbles of resonance with kindred spirits where we are impervious to the darkness of the external chaos and can use it for an evolutionary purpose of liberating ourselves while encouraging one another to thrive.

When we are in the liminal spaces, we start to feel the emergence and arrival of the new, yet we don't really know exactly what it will be until we experience it as it starts to take form.

It is going to be surprising, unexpected, challenging and also *beautiful*!

We are living in wild and pivotal years on planet Earth. I believe that those of us who are alive now were born for these times. Let's ignore the ongoing fear and coercive control attempts to infect us with more victimhood consciousness, rescue fantasies, and captivity.

When in doubt, fear, uncertainty, powerlessness, or self-pity, ask yourself, *how does it serve you*?

This is the evolutionary calling of our lifetime. How we respond as individuals will determine our personal fate, and the sum of our individual choices will become the future of humanity—our legacy.

The legacy you inherited, and your most challenging life experiences, have prepared you for the opportunity to evolve during these times.

What kind of legacy will you pass on?

What will you tell your kids or grandkids in the future about the role you played during this turning point in human history?

I invite you to participate in opening a brighter path for yourself, humanity, and future generations by *becoming whole* and transforming your wounds into a legacy of light.

Your choices create your legacy.

Your choice is your power.

ENDNOTES

[1] National Domestic Violence Hotline, "Supporting Someone Who Keeps Returning to an Abusive Relationship," https://www.thehotline.org/resources/supporting-someone-who-keeps-returning-to-an-abusive-relationship/ (accessed March 11, 2025).

[2] Joseph Murphy, *The Power of Your Subconscious Mind* (Radford, VA: Wilder Publications, 2008).

[3] Rancourt, Denis, and Correlation. "Medical Hypothesis: Respiratory Epidemics and Pandemics without Viral Transmission." Medical Hypothesis: Respiratory Epidemics and Pandemics without Viral Transmission, Denis's Substack, 3 Dec. 2024, denisrancourt.substack.com/p/medical-hypothesis-respiratory-epidemics.

[4] Andrew Huberman, "Science of Social Bonding in Family, Friendship & Romantic Love," YouTube video, 2:15:29, December 20, 2021, https://www.youtube.com/watch?v=RgAcOqVRfYA (accessed June 6, 2025).

[5] N. Leigh-Hunt et al., "An overview of systematic reviews on the public health consequences of social isolation and loneliness," *Public Health*, Vol. 152 (2017), pp. 157–171, https://pubmed.ncbi.nlm.nih.gov/28915435/ (accessed June 6, 2025).

[6] Napoleon Hill, *Outwitting the Devil: The Secrets to Freedom and Success* (Shippensburg, PA: Sound Wisdom, 2020).

[7] Ibid.

[8] Patrick J. Carnes, *The Betrayal Bond: Breaking Free of Exploitive Relationships* (Deerfield Beach, FL: Health Communications, Inc., 2019).

[9] Samantha Murphy Kelly, "Vaccine Selfies Are Everywhere. That's Actually a Good Thing," CNN, March 6, 2021, https://edition.cnn.com/2021/03/06/tech/covid-vaccine-selfie (accessed June 6, 2025).

[10] PressForTruth, "Canadians Now REQUIRED SHOT EVERY 9 MONTHS!" Rumble video, 11:00, 2022, https://rumble.com/v1b8h81-canadians-now-required-shot-every-9-months-you-will-never-be-fully-vaxxed-c.html (accessed June 6, 2025).

11 Natasha Korecki and Christopher Cadelago, "'It's about time': Biden puts the screws on the unvaccinated," *Politico*, September 10, 2021, https://www.politico.com/news/2021/09/10/biden-pandemic-vaccination-effort-511157 (accessed June 7, 2025).

12 "Biden to the unvaccinated: 'Our patience is wearing thin,'" CNN, September 9, 2021, video, https://www.cnn.com/videos/politics/2021/09/09/biden-message-unvaccinated-americans-patience-sot-lead-vpx.cnn (accessed June 7, 2025).

13 Allie Malloy and Maegan Vazquez, "Biden warns of winter of 'severe illness and death' for unvaccinated due to Omicron," CNN, December 16, 2021, https://www.cnn.com/2021/12/16/politics/joe-biden-warning-winter/index.html (accessed June 7, 2025).

14 Meredith Miller, "Weaponized Fear Corrupts the Human Operating System," in C.H. Klotz, ed., *Canary in a (Post) Covid World: Money, Fear and Power*, Vol. 2 (Canary House Publishing, 2024).

15 Melanie B. Tannenbaum et al., "Appealing to fear: A meta-analysis of fear appeal effectiveness and theories," *Psychological Bulletin*, Vol. 141, No. 6 (November 2015), pp. 1178–1204, https://pubmed.ncbi.nlm.nih.gov/26501228/ (accessed June 7, 2025).

16 Robin L. Nabi and Jessica Gall Myrick, "Uplifting Fear Appeals: Considering the Role of Hope in Fear-Based Persuasive Messages," *Health Communication*, Vol. 34, No. 4 (April 2019), pp. 463–474, https://pubmed.ncbi.nlm.nih.gov/29313717/ (accessed June 7, 2025).

17 Google, "Get Back to What You Love," YouTube video, 1:01, March 23, 2021, https://youtu.be/k3y1hJPVavY (accessed June 7, 2025).

18 The Vaccine Confidence Project, "Get Back to What You Love," YouTube playlist, 2021, https://www.youtube.com/playlist?list=PLxtTUK56wH7pJSxRFRUaBDbV0ANBCej_f (accessed June 7, 2025).

19 "Suddenly, Hope," *The Economist*, November 14, 2020, https://www.economist.com/weeklyedition/2020-11-14 (accessed June 7, 2025).

20 Yale University, "COVID-19 Vaccine Messaging, Part 1," ClinicalTrials.gov, Study ID NCT04460703, Completed 2020, https://clinicaltrials.gov/study/NCT04460703 (accessed June 7, 2025).

21 Margaret Anna Alice, "Anatomy of a Philanthropath: Dreams of Democide & Dictatorship," Margaret Anna Alice Through the Looking Glass (Substack), June 24, 2022, http://philanthropaths.com (accessed June 7, 2025).

22 Daniel S. Lobel, "People-Pleasing as a Symptom of Childhood Trauma," *Psychology Today*, August 4, 2024, https://www.psychologytoday.com/us/blog/my-side-of-the-couch/202408/people-pleasing-as-a-symptom-of-childhood-trauma (accessed June 8, 2025).

23 Sharon Kirkey, "Ontario Man Granted Euthanasia for Controversial 'Post COVID-19 Vaccination Syndrome,'" *National Post*, October 24, 2024,

https://nationalpost.com/health/ontario-man-euthanasia-post-covid-19-vaccination-syndrome (accessed June 8, 2025).

24 Margaret Anna Alice, "Mistakes Were NOT Made: An Anthem for Justice," Margaret Anna Alice Through the Looking Glass (Substack), January 1, 2023, http://mistakeswerenotmade.com (accessed June 8, 2025).

25 John Eldredge, *Wild at Heart: Discovering the Secret of a Man's Soul*, Expanded ed. (Nashville: Thomas Nelson, 2021).

26 Ibid.

27 Ibid.

28 Ayn Rand, *Atlas Shrugged*, 1st Signet mass-market ed. (New York: Penguin Random House, 1996).

29 Axel Franzen and Sebastian Mader, "The power of social influence: A replication and extension of the Asch experiment," *PLoS One*, Vol. 18, No. 11 (November 2023), pp. e0294325, https://pmc.ncbi.nlm.nih.gov/articles/PMC10686423/ (accessed June 9, 2025).

30 Ibid.

31 Meredith Miller, "No Is a Complete Sentence…RED FLAGS in the Vaxx Conversation," Rumble video, 2021, https://rumble.com/vrlltd-no-is-a-complete-sentence...-red-flags-in-the-vaxx-conversation.html (accessed June 9, 2025).

32 Blue Seat Studios, "Tea Consent," YouTube video, 2:50, May 12, 2015, https://youtu.be/oQbei5JGiT8 (accessed June 9, 2025).

33 Encyclopedia.com, "Nuremberg Code Establishes the Principle of Informed Consent," https://www.encyclopedia.com/science/medical-magazines/nuremberg-code-establishes-principle-informed-consent (accessed March 11, 2025).

34 "Coercive or controlling behaviour now a crime," Gov.uk, December 29, 2015, https://www.gov.uk/government/news/coercive-or-controlling-behaviour-now-a-crime (accessed June 9, 2025).

35 Ibid.

36 The Jimmy Dore Show, "Yes, People Were Forced to Get the Vaxx!—Australian Politician Tells Pfizer Execs," YouTube video, 14:01, August 8, 2023, https://youtu.be/BBWTBaCqnBQ (accessed June 9, 2025).

37 Ibid.

38 Enlightened Prophetz, "Tony Blair Speaks at WEF 2023," YouTube video, 5:16. January 19, 2023, https://youtu.be/8OKLzfTE8Eg (accessed June 9, 2025).

39 Julian Savulescu and Hilary Bowman-Smart, "Moral Bioenhancement and Future Generations: Selecting Martyrdom?" in Stephen M. Gardiner, ed., *The Oxford Handbook of Intergenerational Ethics*, online edition, March 10, 2021, https://doi.org/10.1093/oxfordhb/9780190881931.013.53 (accessed March 26, 2025).

40 Parker Crutchfield, "Compulsory moral bioenhancement should be covert," *Bioethics*, Vol. 33, No. 1 (2019), pp. 112–121, https://pubmed.ncbi.nlm.nih.gov/30157295/ (accessed June 9, 2025).

41 Andrew Gregory, "Covid vaccine hesitancy could be linked to childhood trauma, research finds," *The Guardian*, February 1, 2022, https://www.theguardian.com/society/2022/feb/01/covid-vaccine-hesitancy-could-be-linked-childhood-trauma-research (accessed June 9, 2025).

42 Mark A. Bellis et al., "Associations between adverse childhood experiences, attitudes towards COVID-19 restrictions and vaccine hesitancy: a cross-sectional study," *BMJ Open*, 2022, https://bmjopen.bmj.com/content/12/2/e053915 (accessed June 9, 2025).

43 Public Health Wales, "Coronavirus vaccine hesitancy linked to childhood trauma," February 2, 2022, https://phw.nhs.wales/news/coronavirus-vaccine-hesitancy-linked-to-childhood-trauma/ (accessed June 9, 2025).

44 Bellis et al., "Associations between adverse childhood experiences, attitudes towards COVID-19 restrictions and vaccine hesitancy: a cross-sectional study."

45 Gregory, "Covid vaccine hesitancy could be linked to childhood trauma, research finds."

46 Ibid.

47 Ibid.

48 Merriam-Webster.com, "Compliance: noun," https://www.merriam-webster.com/dictionary/compliance (accessed March 30, 2025).

49 Jesse Maxwell Kohler, "A Trauma Informed Approach to Vaccine Fear," PACEs Connection, November 5, 2021, https://pacesconnection.crowdstack.io/blog/a-trauma-informed-approach-to-vaccine-fear.

50 Ibid.

51 Aaron Siri, "Why a Judge Ordered FDA to Release Covid-19 Vaccine Data Pronto," Bloomberg Law, January 18, 2022, https://news.bloomberglaw.com/health-law-and-business/why-a-judge-ordered-fda-to-release-covid-19-vaccine-data-pronto (accessed June 9, 2025).

52 Naomi Wolf, "What's in the Pfizer Documents?" Hillsdale College Freedom Library, March 6, 2023, video, https://freedomlibrary.hillsdale.edu/programs/cca-iv-big-pharma/what-s-in-the-pfizer-documents (accessed June 9, 2025).

53 Mary McMahon, "What Was the Tuskegee Experiment?" AmericaExplained.org, May 17, 2024, https://www.americaexplained.org/what-was-the-tuskegee-experiment.htm (accessed June 10, 2025).

54 John W. Oller et al., "HCG Found in WHO Tetanus Vaccine in Kenya Raises Concern in the Developing World," *Open Access Library Journal*, Vol. 4, No. 10 (October 2017), pp. 1–32, https://www.scirp.org/journal/paperinformation?paperid=81838 (accessed June 10, 2025).

55 Shena Cavallo, "Peru: Forced Sterilization of 272,000 Indigenous Women 'Not a Crime Against Humanity,'" The Campaign to STOP GE Trees,

September 13, 2016, https://stopgetrees.org/peru-forced-sterilization-of-272000-indigenous-women-not-a-crime-against-humanity/ (accessed June 10, 2025).

[56] Pew Research Center, "Public Trust in Government: 1958–2024," June 24, 2024, https://www.pewresearch.org/politics/2024/06/24/public-trust-in-government-1958-2024/ (accessed June 10, 2025).

[57] Kohler, "A Trauma Informed Approach to Vaccine Fear."

[58] Natalie Grover, "Children Born During Pandemic Have Lower IQs, US Study Finds," *The Guardian*, August 12, 2021, https://www.theguardian.com/world/2021/aug/12/children-born-during-pandemic-have-lower-iqs-us-study-finds (accessed June 10, 2025).

[59] Megan Redshaw, "1.2 Million Reports of Injuries After COVID Vaccines, VAERS Data Show," *The Defender*, April 29, 2022, https://childrenshealthdefense.org/defender/vaers-vaccine-injuries-covid-shot-cdc-data/ (accessed June 10, 2025).

[60] RVM News, "Died Suddenly: 100+ Headlines from Just 10 Days—Serious Heart Issues & Severe Complications," Rumble video, undated, https://rumble.com/v1qjf5q-died-suddenly-100-headlines-from-just-10-days-serious-heart-issues-and-seve.html (accessed June 10, 2025).

[61] Nuclear Vault, "Duck and Cover (1951) Bert the Turtle," YouTube video, 9:15, July 11, 2009, https://www.youtube.com/watch?v=IKqXu-5jw60 (accessed June 12, 2025).

[62] Robert D. Putnam, *Bowling Alone: The Collapse and Revival of American Community* (New York: Simon & Schuster, 2000).

[63] "Why Haven't We Seen a Photograph of the Whole Earth Yet?" Why Haven't We Seen a Photograph of the Whole Earth Yet? - AR0502 | Busy Beaver Button Museum, buttonmuseum.org/buttons/why-havent-we-seen-photograph-whole-earth-yet. Accessed 16 July 2025.

[64] Fred Turner. "From Counterculture to Cyberculture." University of Chicago Press. May 15, 2008.

[65] Politics and Prose. "Annie Jacobsen, 'Operation Paperclip.'" March 15, 2014. https://youtu.be/HHs5M3pyd3Q?si=PaR-_5dxInHNhcjk.

[66] Danny Lewis. Smithsonian magazine. "Why the U.S. Government Brought Nazi Scientists to America After World War II." November 16, 2016 https://www.smithsonianmag.com/smart-news/why-us-government-brought-nazi-scientists-america-after-world-war-ii-180961110/

[67] NOAA. "Weather Modification Project Reports." Accessed July 14, 2025. https://library.noaa.gov/weather-climate/weather-modification-project-reports

[68] *The Holy Bible*, Majority Standard Bible (MSB), Bible Hub, 2023.

[69] *The Holy Bible*. New King James Version, (Nashville: Thomas Nelson, 1982).

[70] Xiao Liu, "Tracking How Our Bodies Work Could Change Our Lives," World Economic Forum, June 4, 2020, https://www.weforum.org/

agenda/2020/06/internet-of-bodies-covid19-recovery-governance-health-data/ (accessed June 12, 2025).

[71] Rick Mayer, "A Johns Hopkins Study Says 'Ill-Founded' COVID Lockdowns Did More Harm Than Good," *Health News Florida*, February 2, 2022, https://health.wusf.usf.edu/health-news-florida/2022-02-02/a-johns-hopkins-study-says-ill-founded-lockdowns-did-little-to-limit-covid-deaths (accessed June 12, 2025).

[72] Rhoda Wilson. "Covid vaccine mandates for police and ambulance workers were unlawful, an Australian court has found." Feb 28, 2024. https://expose-news.com/2024/02/28/covid-vaccine-mandates-were-unlawful-australia/

[73] Health Freedom Defense Fund Team. "Idaho Leads the Nation with Landmark Medical Freedom Legislation". April 6, 2025. https://healthfreedomdefense.org/idaho-leads-the-nation-with-landmark-medical-freedom-legislation/covid-vaccine-mandates-were-unlawful-australia/

[74] Rasmussen Reports, "COVID-19 Democratic Voters Support Harsh Measures Against the Unvaccinated," January 2022, https://www.rasmussenreports.com/public_content/politics/partner_surveys/jan_2022/covid_19_democratic_voters_support_harsh_measures_against_unvaccinated (accessed June 12, 2025).

[75] Anandamide. "Whole Genome Sequencing of Fibrin Clots." Substack. May 23, 2025. https://anandamide.substack.com/p/whole-genome-sequencing-of-fibrin.

[76] Zohaib Yousaf, Fateen Ata, Riyadh Ali Mohammed Hammamy, "Thrombosis post-mRNA-based SARS-CoV-2 vaccination (BNT162b2) – Time to think beyond thrombosis with thrombocytopenia syndrome (TTS)". April 18, 2022. https://doi.org/10.1016/j.tru.2022.100104. https://www.sciencedirect.com/science/article/pii/S2666572722000086

[77] Sherri Tenpenny, "Welcome to Eye on the Evidence - Starting with Myocarditis: A Discussion on Articles from Peer-Reviewed Literature." Substack. June 12, 2022. https://drtenpenny.substack.com/p/introducing-eye-on-the-evidence

[78] Shifted Paradigm, "Harari: What Do We Do With the Useless Eaters?" YouTube video, 3:00, March 13, 2017, https://www.youtube.com/watch?v=Ex3_brOUdpA (accessed June 12, 2025).

[79] John Bradshaw, *Reclaiming Virtue: How We can Develop the Moral Intelligence to the Right Thing at the Right Time for the Right Reason* (New York: Bantam, 2009).

[80] Ibid.

[81] Ibid.

[82] *The NeverEnding Story*, directed by Wolfgang Petersen (Burbank, CA: Warner Bros., 1984).

ABOUT THE AUTHOR

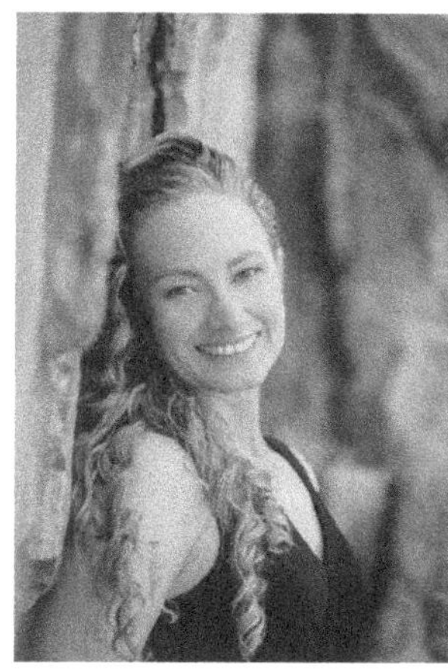

Meredith Miller is a holistic coach, author, and speaker. Her mission is bridging the gap between trauma and purpose. One of the courageous voices in these wild times on planet Earth, Meredith is here to help you evolve and thrive beyond generational trauma and the existential pressure of the 2020s. Meredith is a graduate of the University of Pennsylvania. She helps people transmute the past into gold and transform their wounds into a legacy of light so they can step into their divine purpose and make a difference in the world around them. Meredith is passionate about helping people liberate themselves and evolve so they can live as free, empowered, responsible, awakened, purposeful, and actualized human beings who contribute to the liberation and evolution of others in their own unique ways.